Success in Academic Surgery

Series Editors

Lillian Kao
McGovern School
The University of Texas Health Science Centre
Houston, TX
USA

Herbert Chen
Department of Surgery
University of Alabama at Birmingham
Birmingham, AL
USA

All of the intended volume editors are highly successful academic surgeons with expertise in the respective fields of basic science, clinical trials, health services research, and surgical education research. They are all also leaders within the Association for Academic Surgery (AAS). The previous AAS book, Success in Academic Surgery: Part I provided an overview with regards to the different types of surgical research, beginning one's academic career, and balancing work and life commitments. The aims and scopes of this series of books will be to provide specifics with regards to becoming successful academic surgeons with focuses on the different types of research and academic careers (basic science, clinical trials, health services research, and surgical education). These books will provide information beyond that in the introductory book and even beyond that provided in the Fall and International Courses. The target audience would be medical students, surgical residents, and young surgical faculty. We would promote bulk sales at the Association for Academic Surgery (AAS) Fall Courses (www.aasurg.org) which take place prior to the American College of Surgeons meeting in October, as well as the AAS International Courses which take place year-round in Australasia, Colombia, West Africa, and France. Courses are also planned for India, Italy, and Germany and potentially in the United Kingdom and Saudi Arabia. As the AAS expands the course into other parts of the world, there is a greater need for an accompanying series of textbooks. The AAS has already received requests for translation of the book into Italian. These books would be closely linked with the course content and be sold as part of the registration. In 2011, there were 270 participants in the Fall Courses. In addition, we would anticipate several hundred participants combined per year at all of the international courses.

More information about this series at http://www.springer.com/series/11216

Mark S. Cohen • Lillian Kao
Editors

Success in Academic Surgery: Innovation and Entrepreneurship

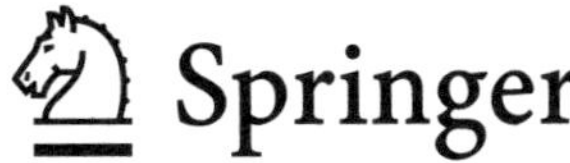 Springer

Editors
Mark S. Cohen
Department of Surgery
University of Michigan
Ann Arbor, MI
USA

Lillian Kao
McGovern School
The University of Texas Health
Science Centre
Houston, TX
USA

ISSN 2194-7481   ISSN 2194-749X   (electronic)
Success in Academic Surgery
ISBN 978-3-030-18612-8   ISBN 978-3-030-18613-5   (eBook)
https://doi.org/10.1007/978-3-030-18613-5

This Springer imprint is published by the registered company Springer Nature Switzerland AG
The registered company address is: Gewerbestrasse 11, 6330 Cham, Switzerland

Contents

Introduction

The relationship between technology and surgery has grown exponentially in the last decade and has become vital to the practice and advancement of the field. As such, surgeons and trainees are inundated with new technologies being applied to their practice every day, and it has become crucial for surgeons to not only understand how these technologies could impact patient care and improve surgical diseases but also how to decide which technologies are the safest, most reliable, and impactful. Additionally, in academic surgery, the mission of advancing the field with translational research, clinical outcomes, and education now must include some interaction with surgical technology and innovations. To be at the forefront of how to improve surgery for patients and treatment of surgical diseases, academic surgeons are tackling today's challenges and problems in surgery using surgical innovations. In fact, many institutions now recognize these academic efforts in innovation and entrepreneurship as a viable outlet for career development and productivity.

Each year more, practicing surgeons and trainees are engaging in the development of novel devices, therapeutics, digital health solutions, and process/policy innovations for the improved care of surgical patients and surgical diseases. With this in mind, and to be at the forefront of surgical science and advances in patient care, it is important for surgeons at all levels to better understand the process of surgical innovation and entrepreneurship and how to develop or apply new technologies more effectively for their patients. This textbook was developed with the goal of helping surgeons and trainees gain a more thorough understanding of the state of the art regarding innovation and entrepreneurship in academic surgery as well as methods to overcome hurdles and challenges in the development and implementation of new surgical technologies. This is a very exciting time for surgeons around the globe to create and apply novel technologies that will have a meaningful impact on the care of surgical patients, and we are pleased to provide you with the most innovative and impactful methods, programs, and processes as a resource on how this can be accomplished in a thoughtful way.

This book is organized to provide the reader with a meaningful overview of the process for developing surgical innovations from concept to commercial product, as well as numerous models within academic surgery where this process has been successful. This includes creating a meaningful value proposition and a compelling pitch, the process of customer discovery; pivoting your idea for a better impact; understanding intellectual property, patents, and conflicts of interest; and navigating the regulatory pathway. The book provides multiple case-based examples of surgical innovations and their journeys through commercialization, whether this resulted in a disruptive technology that improved the field, an important pivot, or a failure where key lessons were learned. We also include a perspective on the importance of industry-academic partnerships, funding models, and the role of education and training medical students, residents, and surgeons in practice in the art of developing successful surgical innovations. We hope this textbook on innovation and entrepreneurship will be an important resource for surgeons and trainees around the world engaging in this exciting and growing area of academic surgery.

Mark S. Cohen, MD, FACS

Lillian Kao, MD, FACS

Chapter 1
Developing a Surgical Innovation: Creating a Meaningful Value Proposition and a Compelling Pitch for Impact

David Olson and Mark S. Cohen

Introduction

Having a good idea and turning it into a meaningful innovation that will positively impact society requires a good understanding of the process of innovation and commercialization. It starts with defining the right problem to address and then brainstorming ideas that solve the problem. Those ideas then need to be tested and evaluated by a variety of stakeholders and customers who can help focus the idea to something that is more valuable to them and has meaningful impact. Once a good idea is crafted into a strong value proposition, it needs resources and the right team to move it forward. Bringing others into your innovation and creating a shared vision to move it through the commercialization process require you to develop skills in giving a compelling pitch. This first chapter provides an overview of the ideation and innovation process as well as helpful insights to guide your medical innovations and prepare you to be more successful in this creative process. We have also included at the end, some links for you to observe how practicing academic surgeons can create compelling pitches of their innovations that can lead to meaningful impact.

D. Olson
Office of Technology Transfer, University of Michigan, Ann Arbor, MI, USA
e-mail: davidols@umich.edu

M. S. Cohen (✉)
Department of Surgery, University of Michigan, Ann Arbor, MI, USA
e-mail: cohenmar@med.umich.edu

© Springer Nature Switzerland AG 2019
M. S. Cohen, L. Kao (eds.), *Success in Academic Surgery: Innovation and Entrepreneurship*, Success in Academic Surgery,
https://doi.org/10.1007/978-3-030-18613-5_1

Important Definitions

Before embarking on the innovation process, it is important to first mention and define some important terminology that often get confused in this space in order to be clear in how to differentiate ideas from innovations from entrepreneurship and commercialization.

Inspiration The process of being mentally stimulated to do or feel something, especially to do something creative.

Idea A thought, concept, or mental suggestion as to a possible course of action or solution to a problem.

An idea is *not* however a sign of creativity. Nor is it synonymous with innovation or a competitive advantage, and no matter how much you might like it to be, an idea is certainly not a business.

Ideation The process of generating and developing ideas.

Innovation The application of better ideas and solutions that meet new requirements, unarticulated needs, or existing market needs.

The main difference between creativity and innovation is the focus. Creativity is about unleashing the potential of the mind to conceive new ideas. Innovation, on the other hand, is a defined and measurable output. Innovation is about introducing change into relatively stable systems or the implementation or actuation of a new idea or the work or process required to make an idea viable.

Entrepreneurship The activity of setting up a business or businesses and taking on financial risks in the hope of profit.

Commercialization The process of introducing a new product or production method into commerce—making it available on the market.

Intellectual Property A work or invention that is the result of creativity, such as a manuscript or a design, to which one has rights and for which one may apply for a patent, copyright, trademark, etc. It is any product of the human intellect that the law protects from unauthorized use by others.

Design Thinking Design thinking is an iterative process for solving complex problems. There are several steps in the process but depending on the problem and what has been done to solve it thus far, these steps do not necessarily have to occur in sequence. Typically, the first step in this process is *empathizing with users that are experiencing the problem*. Understanding the "pain" or issue from their perspective is critical to the process. This process helps the innovator to better understand and *define the real problem to solve* from the user or stakeholder perspective. This understanding of the problem is also termed "customer discovery" and is a pillar of innovative thinking. Understanding the problem or pain from the user's perspective or from multiple stakeholder perspectives allows one to *create new ideas and innovate* to challenge current assumptions more effectively and *develop novel or alternative solutions or prototypes* that solve the problem that may not be obvious from a cursory evaluation on the surface or from one user's perspective. Once prototype solutions for the right problem are identified, these must be *tested* to determine if they actually solve the problem not just for the innovator, but then this must go back to the user or customer with the problem to determine if they feel the solution adequately addresses the pain or problem and if this has value to them. If not, then data obtained from this customer discovery is used to iterate changes to the solution that then need to be retested and re-evaluated by the customer. This is the iterative process that goes into design thinking [1].

Identifying the Right Problem

One of the keys to creating impactful research, innovations, and disruptive technologies is asking the right question and determining the key problems in medicine that innovative technologies can solve. Just because you make something, does not mean people will want it or that it solves an important problem. In fact, one of the main reasons many new devices, drugs, or innovations fail is that they do not solve the problem for the customer in a meaningful way. For this reason, the first step in innovation development must center around understanding what problem you want to solve. Part of this problem analysis should also include the scope of the problem, what has been done already to address the problem, what are the limitations of those solutions, and most importantly – who will really care if you solve this problem?

How do you scope your problem? Putting scope to your problem is important as it helps you not only understand the size of your potential market, but typically the bigger the problem and scope, the more challenging it is to find a single disruptive solution. Conversely if your problem is only something experienced by 100 people in the world, it may be hard to get investors excited about funding something with this small a benefit. This exercise of scoping is useful to help you create a model with some boundaries around what the problem really is and how many people it is impacting. During this scoping process it is also helpful to determine "WHAT" the problem really is for the people affected.

For example, let's say you wish to create a solution for patient compliance with taking medications. While you are scoping this problem you quickly realize that compliance is a problem for millions of people worldwide, but that the reasons for this lack of compliance are very multifactorial and a single solution would not address all the real reasons for non-compliance. In this case you may want to focus your solution on patients who experience non-compliance due to lack of understanding when they need to take their medications and you made decide for this subset of patients from the bigger cohort of non-compliers, the best solution may be an app to remind them when to take their medications. Such a solution may be easier to develop and test in a group where the problem is more specifically understood.

It is extremely helpful therefore if you take the time early on to scope out the problem, do a bit of a root-cause analysis of what is the real problem you want to solve for the customer, and then understanding how big or small a problem is it.

What solutions exist? The next step in the process once you scope a problem is to figure out what if any solutions currently exist to help with the problem and where do they fall short. This exercise is helpful to know what has already failed or why the current solutions are not good enough. This will help you start to develop your competitive advantage as to how your solution could be better than existing technologies and why your solution is something the customers will really want.

Who cares if you solve this problem? Probably the most significant question you need to answer in any innovation is "who will care if I solve this?" Whether it is investors, patients, or stakeholders, you need to understand who is effected by the solution you are proposing. As part of that identification, it is also important to determine whether that effect is positive or negative. For example if you create a new smartphone app that uses the camera and artificial intelligence algorithms to diagnose skin cancers, while it may be a great potential solution and win for primary care physicians and patients to know what a strange skin lesion is, this solution may be looked at negatively by the dermatology community where their practice and billing would be negatively effected by such a technology. Negative influencers can have as great an impact on whether a technology gets to market as positive influencers so it is very important to think about who all your stakeholders are early on when you are determining who cares about your solution. Also it is good to keep in mind that if your solution will need outside investors such as angels or venture capital funding, you need to understand how many people your technology will help and what revenues will be generated from your solution being used in the market as there are specific metrics these investors will require in order to care about funding your innovation.

Brainstorming and Ideation

After deciding on what is the specific problem you want to solve, the next phase of the innovation process is ideation and brainstorming potential solutions. The best brainstorming often involves team-based brainstorming where you can look at the problem from multiple perspectives and lenses. Diversity of team-based brainstorming can add significant value to identifying novel as well as improbable solutions. In many programs these teams often involve physicians, engineers, business experts, IP lawyers, and customers experiencing the problem. At this phase, no idea is a bad one and it is important to look at every angle and possibility. Generating multiple solutions can be helpful to identify weaknesses in each idea and which ideas have the best chance at solving the problem in order to narrow down your solutions to one lead idea with which to move forward.

Concept Hardening and Iterative De-risking

After defining a lead idea, it needs to be put through a series of tests to determine how it will perform at solving the problem for the customer. Feedback during this period will identify additional weaknesses about the technology. This feedback then will often change the solution a bit to better fit the needs of the customer or to overcome a weakness in the solution. With each iterative improvement, the solution should go back to customers to get more feedback to make sure the fixes indeed make the solution even better. This iterative process shores up weaknesses in the solution and "hardens" it to be more resilient to moving forward to market. Innovation concepts that have been hardened in this way are more likely to garner investors and additional stakeholder buy-in.

In addition to customer feedback, the innovation will also need to be evaluated on how it will get to the customer, i.e. how it will get into the market and how it will be used or adopted. This often will require understanding of its regulatory pathway, intellectual property, reimbursement plan, and sales/adoption especially if it is replacing or competing with existing solutions. All of these factors can be difficult to navigate or create hurdles that the innovation must clear to move forward. Identifying these risks or hurdles early is critical in order to understand the cost and steps needs to surmount them as well how these steps will affect the time it will take for the innovation to get to the customer in the market. If the hurdles along the pathway are too costly, too difficult, or too time-consuming, it may mean the technology may not be viable moving forward and failing early is far better in many cases than putting more time, money and resources into something with little to no chance of success. With each of these hurdles that can be overcome or mitigated, the technology becomes less risky or weak from an investment standpoint and instead becomes de-risked and more likely to generate revenues or succeed in the market. As such, the more de-risked an innovation becomes, the higher the chance investors or strategic partners will be interested in it.

How the Build and Use a Value Proposition

With an idea formed, the next action for innovators is to develop a Value Proposition statement and then test it.

What is a Value Proposition?

A Value Proposition is an easily understood statement that puts forth the rationale for an innovation. It is an answer to the questions "why do you want people to change what they do" and "why are you attempting to commercialize a discovery". In its most mature form the Value Proposition is a distillation of the reasons for advancing an innovation, who will care, and why they will be motivated to adopt the innovation. As taught in this course the Value Proposition is written as a single sentence with the following structure:

> Customers have a Problem and the proposed Solution is better than the alternatives resulting in compelling Value

The Value Proposition statement contains four core elements:

- Customer - in this case, Customer is a term of art that is broadly defined and often synonymous with "Stakeholders" -- individuals, groups and institutions that make the decision to use the innovation, or are primarily affected by the decision to use, the innovation. Note that although the party that actually pays for the innovation is definitely a Stakeholder, the concept of Customer in the context of a Value Proposition is typically more inclusive.
- Problem - a description of the situation or behavior that you seek to disrupt. What do you want the Customer to do differently? In some circumstance the Problem is better framed as an Opportunity, wherein the Customer may not perceive that anything is "wrong" but may nonetheless be attracted to a change.
- Solution - this is the change you wish to bring to the Customer. For commercialization is it typically a product or service. However, the use of a Value Proposition as an articulation of the rationale for change applies to any innovation, such as department protocol or organizational behavior.
- Value - this is the benefit to the Customer(s) of adopting the proposed change. Typically, this is expressed as both the magnitude of the benefit (e.g.: "saves 90 minutes per day") and why the benefit is compelling in the face of the Customers' alternatives (e.g.: "cost less than available products"). Note the that the list of alternatives always includes what the Customer does today (status quo), even if the Customer currently ignores the Problem.

How to Use the Value Proposition to Test Assumptions.

In this course innovators are encouraged to think of the Value Proposition as an assertion, not a fact. It is treated as a hypothesis, one that can be critically evaluated and tested. The assignment for the innovator then is to collect the data necessary to convince themselves and others that the Value Proposition statement is true, and that pursuing the innovation would realize the potential of the proposition.

What is Customer Discovery

The primary tool to test the Value Proposition and customer interest is referred to as "customer discovery", which boils down to asking questions. Otherwise known as primary market research, this tool is used to gather data from Customers/

Stakeholders, with emphasis on those Customers who will decide to pay for, or use, the proposed innovation. Customer discovery is used to answer a variety of questions such as:

- Should we pursue this idea?
- Is the idea worth patenting?
- What is the best use, or primary customer for, this innovation?
- Why would a person, company or institution change what they do now and adopt the proposed innovation?

Customer Discovery Techniques

Effective use of customer discovery requires that the innovator succeed at three things:

1. **Ask questions of the right people.** The process for identifying who to research in customer discovery is commonly referred to as Ecosystem Mapping or Stakeholder Mapping. The Stakeholders in an ecosystem (aka market) include those who consume, recommend, pay for, make, sell, compete with, advocate for or regulate a product or service. Mapping starts with a list of all the individuals, groups or institutions that are Stakeholders and their relationship to the proposed product or service.

   Next, Stakeholders can be stratified by two criteria: influence and motivation. Those who pay for a product or service usually rank highest on the axis of influence. Those who will make (or lose) money as a result of adopting a product or service are typically the most motivated to make (or block) change. For example, most surgical equipment (such as a ventilator) is purchased and paid for by hospitals. The hospital then typically has the highest combination of influence and motivation, followed by physicians (who recommend and use the product) and then more distantly by patients (who benefit from the use of the product). The priority target for customer discovery should be those Stakeholders who have the most motivation and influence to use, approve and/or pay for the product or service. In the example of the ventilator, priority should be given to the decision makers at the hospital, and the physicians that influence them.

2. **Ask the right questions.** The goal of customer discovery is to understand how the Stakeholders view the hypothetical Value Proposition, so the right questions are those that will elicit useful answers to unknowns such as:
   - Who are the Customers and how many are there?
   - Do the Customers believe that they have the Problem as defined, and do they see the proposed Solution as acceptable?
   - What do the Customers perceive the benefits of adopting the Solution, and do they consider the magnitude of the Value to be compelling enough to change their behavior?

When considering the <u>content</u> of customer discovery questions it is important to be aware that ultimately Customers are motivated to act based on their perception that the characteristics of the Solution will result in Value. As a result, it is helpful to consider the Features and Benefits of the product or service. Features are the attributes of the offering (e.g.: dimensions, service life, indication, side effects, price), or *what* the Customer buys. Benefits are the outcome for the Customer (e.g.: can make or save money, better quality of life, meet regulatory requirement), or the *reason* the Customer buys. When these criteria are mapped to the Value Proposition, the Features are the attributes of the Solution, and the Benefits combine to form the Value. Innovators are instructed to identify the Features and Benefits of their proposed product or service, and then to ask Stakeholders about those Features and Benefits, as well as the Features and Benefits of whatever the Stakeholders do, or use, now.

In addition to the content, it is important to consider the <u>form</u> of customer discovery questions. The number one tip is to ask open ended questions. Instead of "do you like?", try "why do you like?". Even better is to ask two separate questions: "What about this do you like?" and "what about this do you not like?". Both are open ended questions, but the latter gets to the second most important advice: seek and encourage negative feedback. Most times interviewees will avoid negative suggestions, potentially resulting in biased answers. If you do not ask direct questions to elicit such feedback you may miss opportunities to catch problems early in your process, before they can sink a product or service after launch.

3. **Conduct the interview process effectively.** Customer Discovery is most effective when done as a face-to-face interview, though phone interviews can also be used. There are several tips for conducting a good interview:

    - The interviewer should listen more than they talk. It is OK to talk about your idea in general terms but control the urge to convince or "win over" the interviewee. If your idea is still confidential you can ask about interest in the performance you plan to deliver, as opposed to how you will achieve that performance.
    - It is advisable to craft your questions in advance, as this helps to start the interview on track, and maximize your time with the interviewee. However, the script should be flexible--the best outcome of any interview is to learn things you did not already know, and the interviewer should go off script when the opportunity arises to explore something new and important.
    - Bringing along a partner, if possible, to focus on taking notes (recording is also acceptable to most interviewers upon request). A partner also adds more listening power, allowing the interviewer focuses on completing the objectives of the interviews.
    - Every interview should be captured in a brief written summary, including basic details like who was interviewed (contact info), when, by whom, and a list of notable findings. A collection of these summaries can be very helpful in making the case to support your innovation when it is time to request funding.

- When wrapping up an interview there are two questions the interviewer should include: "What didn't we ask that we should have?" and "Can you recommend anyone one you know who might be willing to answers these types of questions in an interview?". The former is a great catch all and the latter is a good way to extend your network.

A common question from new innovators is "how do I find people to interview"? The answer ranges from friends, family and colleagues (a great place to start, but not enough) to networked contacts via LinkedIn or professional groups. Also check out journals (for authors of related material) and recent conferences in the field (for lists of speakers). Patient advocacy groups are also often willing to help make contacts, especially for early stage, academic-based technology.

Finally, it is also important to consider the relationship between the innovator and the interviewee. To avoid bias and enable negative feedback it is strongly advised to ask questions outside of your circle of friends and colleagues. Although it can be uncomfortable for the new innovator, direct contact with those whom you don't know (i.e.: a "cold call" but more often via email) is unusually effective. Most people want to help make their world a better place, especially when the questions are couched as an effort to understand the potential of an academic discovery.

Summary

The Value Proposition is a concise statement that states the rationale for advancing an innovation. It can be used as a tool to investigate the market's interest in the innovation. The process of customer discovery is essential for collecting data on the validity of the Value Proposition. Mapping the Stakeholders in the ecosystem is a pre-requisite to efficient customer discovery.

Communicating Innovation Communication is a critical component of the innovation process. Learning to distill thoughts to their essence, and then deliver them in clear and concise manner, is useful in most endeavors. In addition, understanding how the innovation community communicates offers insights as to how others (such as investors and customers) think, and the ability to "speak the language" can help your innovation stand out.

There are a handful of commonly used formats for communicating innovation. The most useful are: the elevator pitch, the executive summary, and the "pitch deck "presentation. The characteristics of each are summarized below.

The Elevator Pitch The classic quick pitch, it is an introduction in about 30 seconds, and as such is not intended to be conclusive. Instead the goal is to "hook" the listener and inspire them to ask for more information. To serve its purpose this pitch must be engaging, but necessarily brief and of limited scope. Perfecting a pitch has the side benefit of forcing the innovator to distill and clarify their message.

The pitch is typically delivered in verbal form. Every pitch is different, but there are common components, such as:

- The Problem or Opportunity
- Your proposed Solution
- Customers/stakeholders who will benefit
- The potential Value

The Executive Summary

The Executive Summary is a written document that covers the essential elements of any plan to advance an innovation. The Executive Summary is not just a longer elevator pitch, but instead it must cover many more topics. The expected content of an Executive Summary varies by industry and setting, but there are shared fundamentals. The following is a good fit for most start-ups, and is segmented into eight sections and defined by the major question they answer:

1. **What kind of innovation/business is this?** The topics include the business sector, (e.g.: drugs, devices, diagnostics, health services, digital health, etc.) and the purpose or function of the start-up (does it discover? develop? manufacture? sell?).
2. **What is the "ask"?** List the amount and type of funding that is sought, and the activities and milestones this funding will enable.
3. **What is the Value Proposition?** State your vision, including what problem or opportunity you wish to address, and why now a compelling chance to act. Describe the Customers and their Problem (or Opportunity). In a succinct manner describe the general concept and key features of the proposed Solution. Describe and quantify the potential benefit--why will Customers care? Summarize the economic rationale for the Customer.
4. **What is the market and competition?** Describe the target market, including size, complexity, notable trends. State why the innovation will be compelling to Customers in face of the competition. Summarize how you will bring this to market and include a high-level outline of marketing and sales strategy, or if applicable, your partnering strategy.
5. **What about patents and regulations?** Summarize your intellectual property position (are there patents or applications?). If applicable, briefly describe any regulatory requirements and your plan to meet those requirements. Finally, if the product is not sold direct to consumers but instead is paid for (at least in part) by insurance, briefly describe your plan to secure reimbursement approval.
6. **Who is on the team?** List the key members of the team who are working toward the venture's goals. Identify the leaders and summarize (in a line or two) why are they are a good fit for the venture.

7. **What will be done and when?** Briefly summarize the critical milestones and the timelines for achieving them.
8. How will investors/funders/stakeholders benefit from supporting you?

List how much will it cost to achieve the listed milestones. Describe how the investors/funders will realize a return on their investment.

Tips for Executive Summaries:

- Best length for an executive summary is 1 or 2 pages
- Focus on Why, What, How, When and Who in each section.
- Strive to be precise and short; use as few words as possible.
- Complete sentences are not necessary; bullet points can be easier to read (and write)

The Pitch Deck

A slide-based presentation--commonly referred to as the "pitch deck"--is ubiquitous in entrepreneuring circles. It can be used both to engage an audience and to develop a relationship. Below are guidelines for crafting a quality pitch deck:

- **Content**: In general, the pitch deck should mirror the topics of the Executive Summary. A good rule of thumb is to cover a single idea or topic per slide. It is easier for the audience if you avoid all-text decks and use images, especially when the image itself conveys content. Data, prototypes or mockups are great, but use them sparingly and to make a point. Tables can provide clarity but consume time, so use them with that consideration. Always use easy to read fonts and colors.
- **Length**: Pitch decks should be flexible depending on the time available. A deck for a first meeting or an introduction with a short time window may be 10–12 slides. A good length for a 60 minute appointment is 30 slides because you should expect interruptions, questions and discussion.
- **Format**: Even though it is created to be delivered "live", always assume that your deck will be read by someone who did not see you present it. In fact, it is not uncommon that the first use of a pitch deck is as an email attachment ("please send me a deck or exec summary"). Accordingly, important content must be understandable to a reader, not just a listener.
- **Order of slides**: There are no hard rules on the order of the content but it is helpful for the audience to lead with elements of the Value Proposition. If the team is a particular strength, then it is often used as a early slide. When in doubt go with what makes the presenter most comfortable.
- **Density**: The duration of your presentation is determined by the content, not by the number of slides. You cannot make a presentation fit into a smaller time window by shrinking the font size. Using a few slides with tiny text only makes it tedious;

more slides with fewer words takes no more time to deliver but it makes each point more impactful. To shorten a presentation, you must distill the content, not cram the slides.

Summary

Communicating your vision requires a combination of tools and formats that share one theme--engage the listener and encourage them to ask for additional information. Brevity is critical but can be difficult for innovators who are inherently excited about their vision and all that is possible. Carving your message to its core elements takes effort. The good news is that brevity can bring insight to both the authors and the audience. A brief message is more likely to engage the audience and win you the chance to say more.

Reference and Links

1. Marshall AC. Business Insider, Primed Associates https://www.businessinsider.com/difference-between-creativity-and-innovation-2013-4. Accessed 10 Apr 2013.

Links for Surgical Innovation Pitch Examples

https://medicine.umich.edu/dept/surgery/news/archive/201810/surgical-innovation-prize-development-accelerator-course
https://www.youtube.com/watch?time_continue=5&v=FpbvFe2wh84
https://www.youtube.com/watch?v=eQzcQV6YzOs&feature=youtu.be
https://www.youtube.com/watch?v=jB8_8eFdCu4&feature=youtu.be
https://www.youtube.com/watch?v=ezJ1-GanQZI&feature=youtu.be
https://www.youtube.com/watch?v=YP5tPKtenmI&feature=youtu.be
https://www.youtube.com/watch?v=H_HM-2BwCZE&feature=youtu.be

Chapter 2
Understanding the Impact of Your Innovation: Customer Discovery

Kyle Miller, Jay Pandit, and Sean Connell

Introduction

Innovation within the medical device space involves a complex lengthy process in order to move technology from the benchtop to the patient's bedside. The ultimate reward for the innovator is to commercialize their technology, creating wide scale impact in the healthcare community. Medical device entrepreneurs and "intrapreneurs" at medical device companies must navigate the traditional hurdles of developing a technology in addition to the added risks of regulatory approval and reimbursement. Most investors, companies and "strategics" are willing to accept a degree of risk in the categories of technical, business, regulatory or reimbursement, but never open their investment funds or research budgets for technologies involving risks across all fronts. Our experience in Northwestern University's Center for Device Development (CD2) program (Evanston, IL), the National Science Foundation's (NSF) Small Business Innovation Research Program (SBIR) "Beat-the-Odds" Boot Camp and the CIMIT (Consortia for Improving Medicine with Innovation and Technology; Boston, MA) accelerator program provided our team at Bold Diagnostics the ability to utilize the customer discovery process in order to create a technology we believe will positively impact noninvasive cardiovascular monitoring.

K. Miller (✉) · J. Pandit · S. Connell
Bold Diagnostics, Inc., Chicago, IL, USA
e-mail: kyle@bolddiagnostics.com; jay@bolddiagnostics.com; sean@bolddiagnostics.com

© Springer Nature Switzerland AG 2019

M. S. Cohen, L. Kao (eds.), *Success in Academic Surgery: Innovation and Entrepreneurship*, Success in Academic Surgery,
https://doi.org/10.1007/978-3-030-18613-5_2

Business Model Canvas

Steve Blank and Bob Dorf's "The Startup Owner's Manual" served as our team's foundational basis as four innovation fellows came together in Northwestern University's Center for Device Development (CD2) program [1]. We utilized Blank and Dorf's Business Model Canvas to organize our early conversations and observations in the cardiovascular space. Further, we modified the canvas so that it was more custom tailored for the medical device arena with a central focus on the unmet clinical need being addressed by the company we formed (Fig. 2.1).

Early Customer Discovery

As Blank and Dorf explain in their book, thirty customer and user interviews should be performed early in the technology development process in order to help guide iterations of the innovation. Ideally, this is done with crude prototypes while the blueprint or business model canvas is still in rough draft format. As an architect looks to transform a client's vision for a home into a foundational structure, a seasoned professional would be the first to admit that a decision to place a front door on the blueprint is much cheaper to change with a pencil and eraser instead of physically reconstructing and moving that door after the home is completed. Admittedly, this process is more logical and easier to utilize for software based technologies; however, our group found the process of customer and user interviews to be immensely useful so that we truly understood the unmet clinical need that we decided to focus on in blood pressure monitoring. Through a series of interviews with nurses, physicians, administrators and patients at Northwestern Memorial Hospital and clinics (Chicago, IL), we were able to determine that existing blood pressure cuff technology suffers from a number of issues including singular discrete measurements, inaccuracies with measurements, poor adherence to positioning requirements, variation in patient anatomy and cuff sizes, etc. The business model canvas we utilized allowed

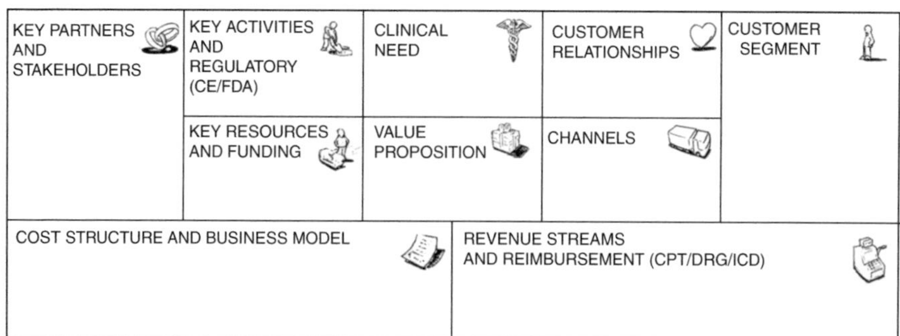

Fig. 2.1 Medical device business model canvas

us to develop the assumptions for the creation of our technology and business. Customer discovery then forced us to leave the confines of our CD2 office and interview users and customers in order to better understand the problem we were solving and the real-life issues of blood pressure monitoring. Further, we uncovered through this initial customer discovery process that patient satisfaction and comfort for patients during their hospital stay was a key problem that the hospital was aware of.

NSF "Beat-the-Odds" Boot Camp Customer Discovery

Our team of innovation fellows formed a limited liability corporation (LLC) once we developed a novel technology for measuring blood pressure non-invasively. After submitting a compelling NSF Phase I grant, we were award non-dilutional funding to further our technology based on promising data generated from an engineering prototype. Phase I grant awardees are then given the option to participate in the NSF "Beat-the-Odds" Boot Camp. The Boot Camp is run twice a year and requires thirty prospective customer interviews. At this point in our technology process, we were able to utilize the Boot Camp to test a number of assumptions we had developed about our customer, physicians dealing with blood pressure management. Although we initially assumed that cohort of physicians was limited to cardiologist and primary care physicians, we learned through the Boot Camp process that our technology had an even broader applicability for OB/GYNs monitoring pre-eclampsia, nephrologist managing complex hypertensive and patients undergoing dialysis, transplant surgeons monitoring their newly transplanted kidney patients along with neurologist monitoring patients at high risk for stroke. Our engineers were able to use rapid prototyping and 3D printing to generate mockups so that we could produce visual aids during our customer discovery process (Fig. 2.2). Further, rapid prototyping was then utilized to create a killer experiment (the type of experiment that is a big go/nogo decision point for a technology) for data generation needed to demonstrate feasibility, proof-of-concept and clinical utility (Fig. 2.3).

Fig. 2.2 Rapid prototyping visual aid

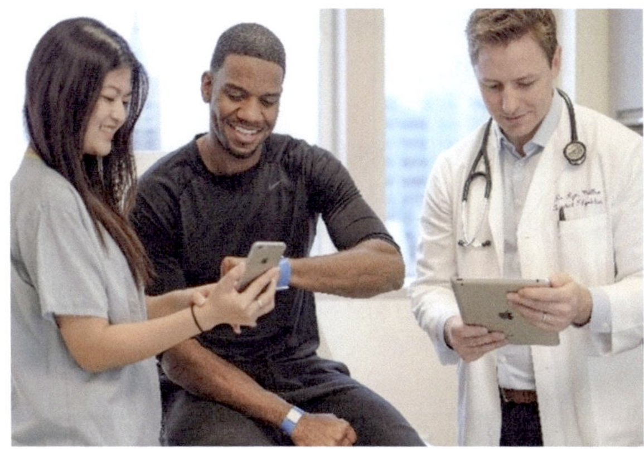

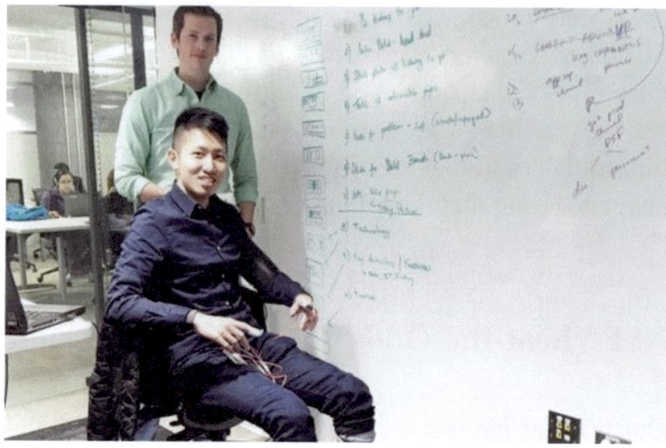

Fig. 2.3 Prototyping testing

We found that pictures of the rapid prototypes and storyboarding helped physicians visualize the potential product and project its potential use into their everyday workflow. Prior experiences taught us that physicians struggled to mentally understand the technology concepts we proposed from a technical standpoint and that a visual aid was absolutely necessary for their analysis of our idea.

There were a number of key stakeholder values from this customer discovery process that we learned during the Boot Camp:

- Usability of existing monitors and feedback on prototypes including form factor
- Existing interruptions and inefficiencies in workflow with blood pressure monitoring protocols
- Clear market segments and physician customer needs
- Distribution channels and decision maker analysis for both inpatient procurement groups and outpatient clinics
- Costs and market willingness for replacing existing devices
- Ideal monitoring period for clinical decision making

CIMIT Stakeholder Discovery and Assumption Funnel Development

Following the NSF Boot Camp, our company elected to participate in the CIMIT (Consortia for Improving Medicine with Innovation and Technology) CRAASH accelerator course. Over the course of several weeks, our company performed ten interviews with various stakeholders to cover ten topics through a customer discovery process:

1. Solution, Product and Service
2. Customer and Value Chain
3. Revenue Model and Potential
4. Validation, Approvals, and Killer Experiment

5. Competitive Understanding and Position
6. Business Protection (IP, etc)
7. Business Economics
8. Go to Market Plan
9. Management Team
10. Capital Needs (Immediate/Total) and Use

Whereas previous customer discovery efforts had our startup and innovation fellows solely focused on customers and users, the CIMIT course challenged the team to focus on stakeholders and truly test major assumptions within the business model canvas. There was a large amount of noise the team had to filter as we heard a vast array of feedback once we began to interact and interview distributors, value analysis committees, operation and commercialization personnel at hospitals, legal experts, business experts in the cardiovascular arena, and investors. We developed the ability over the course of ten weeks and one hundred discussions to develop a solid assumption funnel allowing us to advance toward a formidable business plan while staying lean in our development process. We formulated a considerable value proposition around our technology through three key components during the CRAASH course: cost, comfort, and care. The group did receive some important negative feedback on several key assumptions in our business model that allowed us to rapidly pivot toward a more viable solution for market entry. At this point in our customer and stakeholder interviews, we went from gaining very broad open-ended feedback to capturing our data in quantifiable metrics. This helped inform our market requirement documentation (MRD) as we went from rapid prototyping to a minimum viable product (MVP) that is currently being prepared for regulatory submission and post market clinical studies.

Lessons on Customer Discovery

Ultimately, our innovation team and eventual startup company amassed more than one hundred and sixty customer and stakeholder interviews during our three experiences. We realized through the informative process that stakeholder input is essential. Customer discovery is an essential component of many business accelerator programs and is an essential pillar of both the SBIR and I-CORP business development curricula. The authors highly recommend the business model canvas (Fig. 2.1) to rapidly iterate on ideas and formulate sound assumptions that influence the business plan for the company.

Reference

1. Blank and Dorf. The Startup Owner's Manual: The Step-by-Step Guide for building a Great Company: K & S Ranch; 2012.

Chapter 3
The Center for Innovation in Neuroscience and Technology: A Model for Effective Creativity in Academic Neurosurgery

Eric C. Leuthardt

Abbreviation

CINT   Center for Innovation in Neuroscience and Technology

Introduction

There is currently an acceleration in the emergence of new scientific insights and technical capabilities. Whether one considers computing, biotechnology, imaging, mobile phones, or cloud computing, each innovation makes further technical advances more likely and more efficient. Akin to these general trends, the field of neurological surgery has seen similar dramatic changes in its technical capability. Examples include the emergence of devices for neuromodulation, stereotactic navigation, focused radiation, minimally invasive surgical techniques, novel spinal instrumentation, and a diversity of biologics [1–5]. Today, modern society and medicine are living on an exponentional curve. These rapidly changing dynamics are making it increasingly challenging to stay abreast of the existing knowledge. Moreover, as information continues to expand at an exponential rate, it is becoming harder to predict the future based on the present. This is due to the manner in which we linearly project the future from the present, while the actual pace of change occurs in a non-linear fashion. This pace of scientific and technical change creates new opportunities and challenges for academic medicine to adapt and to continue to provide excellent care.

E. C. Leuthardt (✉)
Department of Biomedical Engineering, Washington University, St. Louis, MO, USA

Department of Neurological Surgery, Washington University School of Medicine,
St. Louis, MO, USA

Department of Neurologic Surgery, Center for Innovation in Neuroscience and Technology,
Washington University School of Medicine, St. Louis, MO, USA
e-mail: leuthardte@wustl.edu

© Springer Nature Switzerland AG 2019
M. S. Cohen, L. Kao (eds.), *Success in Academic Surgery: Innovation and Entrepreneurship*, Success in Academic Surgery,
https://doi.org/10.1007/978-3-030-18613-5_3

Increasingly, it is not possible for an individual to be wholly expert in all the clinical, technical, and scientific aspects that are pertinent to a particular biomedical topic. The model of the individual researcher who incrementally advances an area of medicine is changing to one that is more synergistic. Namely, the incorporation of multiple domains of expertise (both medical and non-medical) are not only critical in the creation of novel scientific and technical insights, but absolutely essential in its translation to clinical application. The synergistic model posits that a multidisciplinary team approach is more effective in performing disruptive research and will be more efficient in achieving necessary milestones for clinical translation. Importantly, this synergistic model incorporates not only technical fields (e.g. medicine, science, and engineering), but also requires fields such as legal, corporate, and financial expertise. Thus, by having collaborators with very different core domain expertise, each of the members can be made more "situationally aware" of the discoveries, technical innovations, and governmental/business trends that can come to bear on a particular research or medical need. Thus, in an era of rapid expansion of human knowledge, the group is better equipped to prepare for the future than is any individual.

Beyond the challenges of staying current, academic neurosurgery (and other technically oriented specialties) faces additional challenges unique to the field. Generally speaking, advances in the practice of neurosurgical care have been driven by the creation of new technologies. However, there are numerous barriers that prevent a neurosurgeon from contributing to this ongoing need for new devices [6]. First and foremost, there is a growing complexity to the innovative process that is in part driven by regulatory and financial developments. Beyond coming up with the good idea, the trained neurosurgeon often has little knowledge of the necessary next steps for advancing an idea from concept to clinical application. Little is taught during neurosurgery residency on necessary steps of idea development and cost of intellectual property, start-up financing, and regulatory hurdles. Thus, a clinician is often faced with a large and seemingly impenetrable ignorance on how best to assess the worth of an idea and how to proceed in validating, protecting, financing, and clinically testing the idea once it has been conceived. Additionally, there is also an inherent challenge in the very earliest stages of exploration when one transitions from a scientific finding to a clinically relevant technology. When financing the translation of scientific discovery to clinical application, there is a transition between government-sponsored research (e.g. National Institute of Health, (NIH)) to private investment (e.g. Venture Capital) as the concept is converted into a product to be sold. That transition is often termed the ***"Valley of Death,"*** from a financing standpoint. This is in part because translational development is less amenable to classic NIH funding, but is too early and risky from an investor standpoint of having a demonstrable product that merits investment. This Valley of Death is often bridged by "Angel Investors"-- regional development agencies, philanthropy, and university technology transfer funds -- and to a more limited degree with NIH grant mechanisms (e.g. Small Business Innovation Research or SBIR, Small Business

Technology Transfer or STTR programs). Finally, there are also challenges within departmental dynamics that further hamper the academic mission. In an environment of declining medical reimbursement and higher operating costs, the classical financial and temporal largesse available for scientific, educational, and innovative pursuits are diminishing. Taken together, though scientific and technical innovation is changing in an exponential manner, it is becoming increasingly difficult for academic surgery to capitalize on these changes due to limitations in access to various domains of expertise, funding barriers in early device development, and a decline in departmental resources to put towards foreword thinking ideas.

In an effort to engage these changing societal dynamics, the Center for Innovation in Neuroscience and Technology (CINT) was created. Fundamental to CINT's mission is the premise that successful creation and translation of innovative ideas rely on the collaboration between multiple disciplines of expertise. From this notion, the CINT has created a unique academic model that integrates scientific, medical, engineering, legal and business domain experts to participate in the full continuum from idea generation to clinical application. By integrating across disciplines, there is an enhanced capability for "effective creativity" within an academic neurosurgical department. Namely, this capability includes an improved ability to generate a higher number of innovative ideas, a more informed perspective to evaluate a concept's clinical and market impact, and an extremely efficient and robust mechanism to generate early stage prototypes to assess the feasibilty of the emergent techologies. By participating, this integrated model also serves to educate and better enable the members of the CINT to engage the demands of a rapidly changing future. This manuscript details the method by which this model has been implemented in the Department of Neurological Surgery at Washington University in St. Louis and the experience that has been accrued thus far.

Mission and Overview

As mentioned, successful advances or innovations in surgical and neuro-related technologies rely on the ongoing interaction between the fields of medicine, engineering, science, law, and business. Building on this premise, the CINT has three core goals that drive its structure and operation: (1) creation of a collaborative environment for the development of novel neuro-medical technologies and facilitation of their real world application; (2) creation of a multidisciplinary education for staff and students to better understand the process of idea generation, valuation, development, and application; and (3) creation of a connection between academia and industry in a mutually beneficial relationship for developing neuro-medical technologies.

The processes of the CINT are created to enable this cross-disciplinary interaction, both within an academic center and between the academic environment and industry. The CINT's process has four fundamental steps (Fig. 3.1). The first step

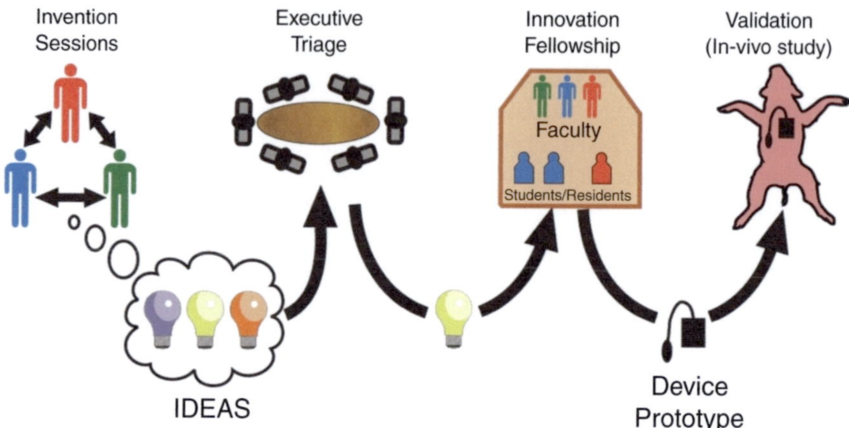

Fig. 3.1 Overview of CINT Process. The figure shows the workflow of idea generation and development within the CINT. There are four potential steps. (1) The "Invention Session" which consists of a structured exchange between physicians, engineers/scientists, and industry representatives. (2) The ideas that are generated across a multitude of Invention Sessions are then collated and triaged by an "Executive Committee" consisting of university leadership across multiple departments and offices. (3) The ideas that are thought to have the highest clinical and market impact and deemed patentable are then sent on to an industry-sponsored multidisciplinary fellowship consisting of neurosurgical and engineering faculty and trainees/students. (4) Top devices felt where further validation is needed are then sent on for in-vivo animal validation studies

and a cornerstone to the CINT is the "Invention Session." These sessions consist of a structured exchange between physicians, engineers/scientists, and industry representatives. This process invariably generates a number of ideas that are documented and catalogued. The ideas that are generated across a multitude of Invention Sessions are then collated and triaged by an "Executive Committee" consisting of university leadership across multiple departments and offices. The ideas that are thought to have the highest clinical and market impact and deemed patentable are then sent on to an industry-sponsored multidisciplinary fellowship consisting of neurosurgical and engineering faculty and trainees/students. The fellowship is an intensive experience focused on creating a functioning prototype of the triaged idea. Once created, the prototypes are then presented to the industry sponsors for corporate feedback. Again, after the creation of multiple prototypes, top devices felt to have the highest promise are then sent on for in-vivo animal validation studies. At the conclusion of this process the CINT is able to provide technologies that have a high potential for translational success. They have been vetted clinically through multiple neurosurgeons. The concepts have protectable intellectual property, have working prototypes available for review, and when necessary, are able to demonstrate in-vivo data in an animal models to support their potential in a clinical trial. All these elements make CINT-produced technologies attractive for industry to license and develop toward devices that are used clinically and sold in the marketplace.

Invention Sessions

The Invention Sessions are one of the cornerstones that the center is built on. These sessions regularly bring together people who do not normally interact: surgeons, engineers, basic scientists, and industry representatives. The Invention Session has a defined three-fold structure in which the inventors agree ahead of time to participate. In the first stage, there is the initial meeting of 4–8 participant inventors. At a minimum, there must be at least two physicians and two engineers/scientists. In this meeting, there will be an exchange between physicians and scientists/engineers in which engineers will discuss their technical capabilities and emerging scientific/technical insights, while the clinicians discuss their practice and the problems and obstacles that they confront on a routine basis. Additionally, when an industry representative is present, that member will also provide insights into what are the important market opportunities that companies are pursuing at present. The goal of the meeting is to create new and innovative technical solutions to improve the practice of neurosurgical and neuro-interventional care of patients.

There are quarterly Invention Sessions that rotate with regards to the members. Currently there are six teams that are driven along clinical themes: vascular, tumor, functional/neurophysiology, spine/orthopedic, trauma/Alzheimer's, and critical care/anesthesia. Groups are chosen based on complementary and/or synergistic skill sets of their members (e.g. vascular surgeon and mechanical engineer). Thus far, faculty from Departments including Neurological Surgery, Vascluar Surgery, Neurology, Anesthesia, Neuro-radiology, Obstetrics and Gynecology, Orthopedics, the School of Engineering (Departments of Biomedical Engineering, Mechanical Engineering, Computer Science), and other neuroscience-relevant domains have been invited to participate.

Executive Triage

The ideas generated across the multiple Invention Sessions are then collated and passed on to the "Executive Committee." The Committee consists of university leadership including the CINT Director; Chairmen of the Departments of Neurosurgery, Biomedical Engineering, and Mechanical Engineering; faculty from Radiology (Neuro-Interventional); the head of the Office of Technology Management; the lead intellectual property attorney from the Office of General Counsel; and a representative from our lead industry sponsor (Stryker Corporation). Together, the group evaluates the high-ranked ideas from the Invention Sessions (across all themes) then rank orders them in terms of priority of development based on the specific criteria. (See Fig. 3.2) The top ideas are then elected to proceed towards prototype validation through the Innovation Fellowship mechanism. This step provides an important triage, in addition to that provided by the inventors, to ensure an added level of objective evaluation separate from the emotional investment that inventors often have associated with their ideas.

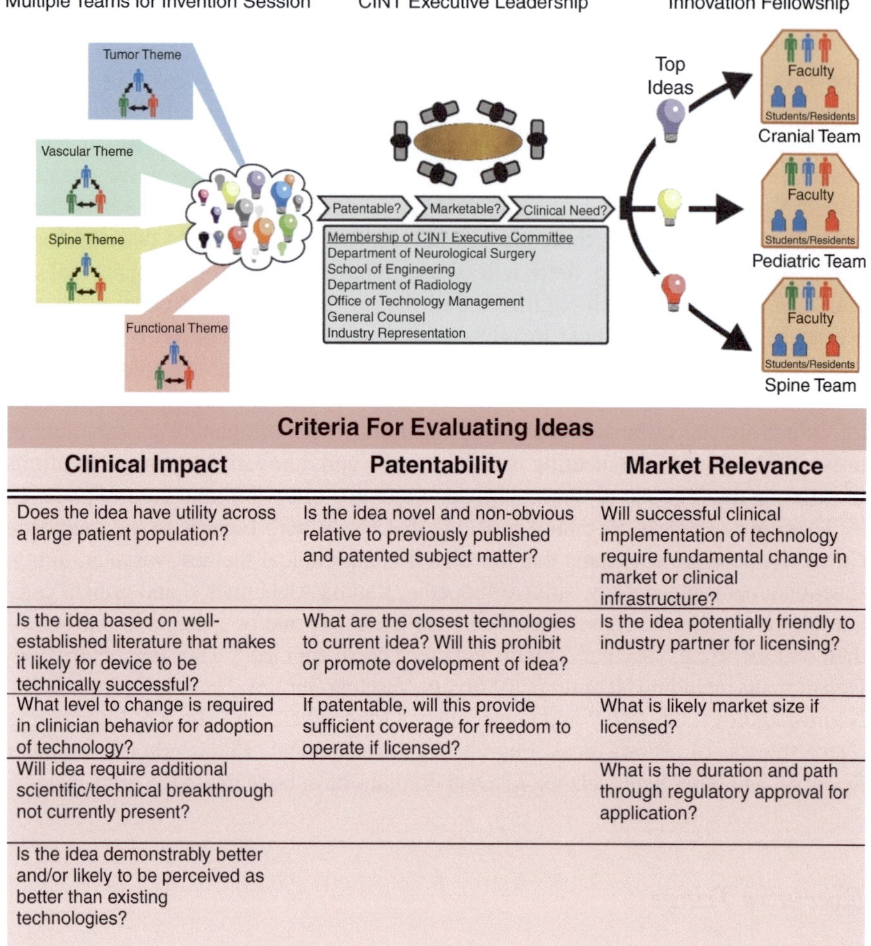

Criteria For Evaluating Ideas		
Clinical Impact	**Patentability**	**Market Relevance**
Does the idea have utility across a large patient population?	Is the idea novel and non-obvious relative to previously published and patented subject matter?	Will successful clinical implementation of technology require fundamental change in market or clinical infrastructure?
Is the idea based on well-established literature that makes it likely for device to be technically successful?	What are the closest technologies to current idea? Will this prohibit or promote dovelopment of idea?	Is the idea potentially friendly to industry partner for licensing?
What level to change is required in clinician behavior for adoption of technology?	If patentable, will this provide sufficient coverage for freedom to operate if licensed?	What is likely market size if licensed?
Will idea require additional scientific/technical breakthrough not currently present?		What is the duration and path through regulatory approval for application?
Is the idea demonstrably better and/or likely to be perceived as better than existing technologies?		

Fig. 3.2 Executive Triage and Criterion for Evaluation of Ideas. The ideas generated across the multiple Invention Sessions are then collated and passed on to the "Executive Committee." The Committee consists of university leadership. Together the group evaluates the high ranked ideas from the Invention Sessions (across all themes) then rank orders them in terms of priority of development based on the specific listed criteria. The top ideas are then elected to proceed towards prototype validation through the Innovation Fellowship mechanism. This step provides an important added layer of triage to supplement the evaluation provided by the inventors and ensure the most objective assessment possible

Innovation Fellowship

A core component of the educational and technical output of the CINT involves the Innovation Fellowship. The fellowship is a unique team-oriented effort that involves both faculty and trainees from the departments of neurosurgery and engineering. It serves the dual role of creating real-world prototypes that can validate the feasibility of a concept and also provides an experience of intense cross-disciplinary interaction that can educate all the participants on the necessary ingredients required for successful ideation and technical translation. At the end of the experience, physicians are more facile at discussing engineering, legal, and industry related issues, while engineers have an improved appreciation for clinical nuance.

Procedurally, after being triaged according to likelihood for clinical success, highly ranked ideas generated from the Invention Sessions are then turned over to an "Innovation Fellowship Team." The team consists of a neurosurgical faculty, an engineering faculty, a neurosurgical resident, and three undergraduate engineering students. The team is then tasked to turn that concept into a working prototype. This involves three milestone steps (Fig. 3.3). The first stage will involve establishing the clinical and medical specifications for the device. The second stage will involve creating the engineering design and draft of the device. The third stage will involve creation of a working physical prototype. A neurosurgical faculty and an engineering faculty oversee each stage. This is a very intense process spanning the spring and summer. Engineering students and neurosurgery residents work together closely to effectively design and implement a prototype that will work and meets the specifications of the neurosurgical faculty. Inclusive in this experience, the fellows will receive multiple lectures from areas of law, finance, and business to better understand the various stages of idea development. The fellowship is then presented to the industry sponsor of the fellowship. Yearly, there are a minimum of five teams -- three during the summer and two during the academic year. Generally, during the

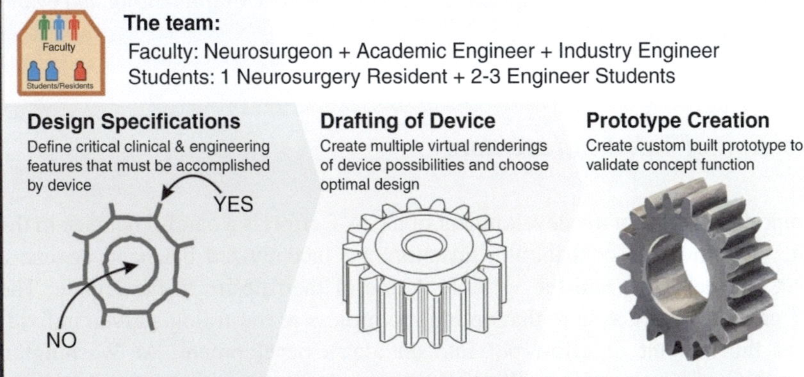

Fig. 3.3 Innovation Fellowship. The fellowship is a team-oriented effort that involves both faculty and trainees from the departments of neurosurgery and engineering. It serves the dual role of creating real world prototypes that can validate the feasibility of a concept, and also provides an experience of intense cross disciplinary interaction that can educate the participants on the necessary steps for successful ideation and technical translation. There are three steps to the fellowship. The first stage will involve establishing the clinical and medical specifications for the device. The second stage will involve creating the engineering design and draft of the device. The third stage will involve creation of a working physical prototype. The prototype is then presented to the industry sponsor of the fellowship

summer session, the teams are broken up into three general themes: a cranial team, a spinal team, and a pediatric team.

Validation Studies

On average, approximately three to five devices are created per year through the Innovation Fellowship mechanism. Again, through criteria similar to the initial screen of ideas at the executive committee, these same filters are applied to the now developed prototypes. The prototypes are additionally evaluated in several ways. First, the experience of creating the device is reviewed. Additional questions as to the device's success in doing what it was originally intended to do and any new unexpected pitfalls with regard to creating the device that could negatively impact the scalability of the device are reviewed. Second, the input from the industry sponsor with regard to market opportunity is taken into consideration. Third, the next steps for the device's translation are projected. Some devices need no further development. In these cases, invention disclosures are submitted to the Office of Technology Management and the devices are actively marketed to both the sponsor and other potential licensees (e.g. device manufactures and venture capital groups). Other devices, to achieve a level of serious consideration for either industry licensing or governmental grant support (e.g. NIH), require further proof of concept in animal models. For those devices that require further development, the CINT works in conjunction with the Department of Comparative Medicine and Veterinary Surgical Services which has large animal facilities capable of implanting and evaluating medical grade devices.

Allocation of Value to Inventors

An important aspect in the development of a CINT effort is a careful balance in the manner in which the contributing inventors are incentivized balanced against a respect for their time and the variable nature of their desire to participate. The CINT created a point system that optimizes fairness in rewarding a given individual for the amount of effort put into an idea's development. At Washington University in St. Louis, the Intellectual Property Policy covers the distribution of net income from license agreements: 35% to inventor(s), 40% to inventor(s) school(s), and 25% to the Office of Research and Office of Technology Management (http://otm.wustl.edu/forfaculty/intellectualproperty.asp). The 35% that is allocated to the faculty participating in the CINT process for a given idea will be subdivided according to a point system based on the how far along the inventor participates in its development. For a given idea, there are several stages involved in its development. These include the following: (1) two meetings for a standard invention session, (2) drafting of the invention disclosure, (3) drafting a design of prototype, (4) creation of prototype, and (5) drafting of a patent. Each of these stages involves a point allocation for a given milestone of accomplishment totaling a certain number of points. For each task beyond the invention session, one or more faculty can participate and thus share in the point allocation for a given milestone. As the tasks are accomplished, the respective points will be assigned to the participating faculty. At the time of the license, the given faculty members' percentage of the 35% allocated to inventors are determined by their number of points divided by the total. Taken together, this allows for a given inventor to balance his or her level of interest against how much they would like to potentially get back. For those who simply enjoy the creative process of inventing, but do not wish to participate in development, they will be rewarded. That reward, however, will be less than that for a co-inventor who works for the coming years to see the idea through the necessary steps of translation.

Inventor Composition and Statistics on Idea Development

Data was taken between the years of 2009 and 2018 during which the CINT's model of idea development has been fully operational. During that time there have been a myriad of inventors across a multitude of disciplines. The group of inventors are broadly divided into two categories – neuroclinical and engineering (79 total). Inventors included faculty from the departments of neurosurgery (13), biomedical engineering (14), mechanical engineering (6), vascular surgery (5), neurology (4), anesthesiology (4), electrical engineering (4), obstetrics and gynecology (3), plastic surgery (2), and computer science. There were also representatives from the office of technology management and industry (15).

There were a total of 48 invention sessions. After triage there were 28 concepts that led to Innovation Fellowship teams. The teams consisted of a total of 95 fellows (28 neurosurgery residents, and 67 engineering students). After completion of these fellowships, there were 37 prototyped concepts that merited invention disclosure to the Office of Technology Management. Nineteen of these concepts were awarded patents. Eleven patents were licensed to companies.

Financial Status

Funding for the CINT has grown 360% since its inception in 2009. The majority of financial support (85%) has come in the form of industry sponsored grants, predominantly from larger medical device manufacturers. Additional support (15%) has come in the form of institutional and regional support for early stage device development.

Discussion

In the highly device-driven fields such as surgery, technical innovation and leadership in the academic mission are largely synonymous. The tenets of leadership in academic surgery revolve around providing cutting edge clinical care, advancing an understanding of topics relevant to the specialty, and training leaders who are capable of producing advances in the field. In both the clinical and research realm, however, this academic mission is threatened secondary to reduced time and finances available to support it. In an environment of declining resources, the classical financial and temporal largesse available for academic pursuits are diminishing. Thus, looking into the future, to maintain the viability of "academic neurosurgery," a department must be able to capture novel revenue streams that will allow its member neurosurgeons to have more free time to do research, teach, and innovate.

The solution to this challenge of actualizing the academic mission while at the same time maintaining a neurosurgical department's financial stability lie in capitalizing on emerging neuro-technology markets through innovative technical solutions. Neurosurgery acts to a large extent as the output arm for a significant portion of neuroscience and engineering applications to patient care. Recent examples of this can be seen with the use of deep brain stimulation in the treatment of depression with targets that have been newly identified with functional imaging [7]. There are currently several thousand practicing neurosurgeons and a smaller fraction of them are academic. This is a small number when considered against the size of the projected neurosurgical device market. The ability to engage these emerging trends in technology and adapt them to neurosurgical needs enables a department to play a leadership role in developing novel medical therapies, while also generating a new source of revenue. This new insight allows a given department to leverage, in a novel way, the expertise it already has. To develop technologies (which neurosurgeons have a unique insight into) that have market value allows a given department to generate revenue from licensing fees and spin off companies that ensue. Since the neurosurgical and neuro-interventional markets are poised for significant growth; this becomes increasingly relevant to the future of these fields.

The CINT model attempts to address some of the translational challenges that currently exist in the current structure of academic and clinical environments. Physicians and engineers face many obstacles in their current working environment in pursuing creative ideas. Their first and most substantial impediment is often a fundamental ignorance to the innovative process. Physicians are rarely well versed in the necessary steps needed to take an idea to practical market application, while the engineer often lacks insight as to where a given technology can be clinically applied. Creating a regularly scheduled interaction between physicians, scientists, engineers, and businessmen in the form of an invention sessions enables each of the members to be more broadly educated, and collectively the group has a knowledge base that overcomes any of the individual's deficits. There are practical time constraints in which participation in the more speculative innovative process detracts from one's more pragmatic professional and financial productivity. Namely, if a surgeon wishes to create a new technology and work towards translating that to a successful industry adoption, this requires a substantial amount of time and financial resources that could otherwise be dedicated to well defined value generating activities (e.g. more cases, industry consulting, legal consulting, etc.). Moreover, because developing new technologies are inherently risky, there is also the possibility that the physician could waste his or her time, thus creating a real opportunity cost. The CINT is structured so that inventing is easy, and subsequent development is organized and supported such that the physician can participate to the level that they are capable. Thus, the burden of development is not solely on a single inventor and thus the price in their time and effort is lower, making them more likely to collectively participate. Finally, the academic and medical culture for the physician and engineer can be inhospitable to creativity in that it often does not support trial and error thinking (poor failure tolerance), entrepreneurial activity, or collaborative enterprise. In the context of the Innovation Fellowship, trial and error and multipronged approaches are an embedded part of the development process. With regard to creating a technical solution, the notion is to fail frequently and quickly until an option can be identified that passes all domains of expertise (e.g. clinically and technically feasible, patent protectable, and good market niche). Thus, in this context it is OK to make mistakes. This is critical for early-unrestrained creative thinking.

In conclusion, the CINT provides a unique model within academic neurosurgery that facilitates the creation of a high number of device-related ideas and facilitates their development in the earliest and most vulnerable stages. The novelty of this model is based on the integrated approach in which multiple domains of expertise are engaged from the moment of an idea's conception through its development at an academic institution. This engagement of cross-disciplinary interaction, early and continuously, leads to synergistic ideas and efficiencies in development that would not have been possible from any of the members alone. Moreover, the experience provides a rich education for the participants on all aspects of ideation and translation. Thus far, the CINT has been successful in generating neuro-technologies that merit industry licensing . If successful in the long term, this innovative institutional approach will stand to improve care of neurosurgical patients by providing new devices that aid in the treatment of their disease and allow neurosurgical departments to have a new revenue stream by effectively and ethically participating in the growing neurosurgical device market.

Acknowledgements I would like to thank Dr. Ralph Dacey for his foresight and vision in supporting this effort. I would also like to thank Stryker Corporation, specifically John Lauria, Matt Powell, and Rick Burmiester, for their vision, patience, and ongoing support in our growing effort at the CINT.

Disclosures and Conflicts of Interest EC Leuthardt holds stock in Neurolutions, Osteovantage, Face to Face Biometrics, Pear Therapeutics, eQuility, Inner Cosmos, Immunovalent.

Funding and Support Stryker Corporation; Bear Cub Fund; Johnson and Johnson; Biogenerator; Ascension Health Ventures.

References

1. Tierney TS, Sankar T, Lozano AM. Deep brain stimulation emerging indications. Prog Brain Res. 2011;194:83–95.
2. Grunert P, Darabi K, Espinosa J, Filippi R. Computer-aided navigation in neurosurgery. Neurosurg Rev. 2003;26(2):73–99; discussion 100-1
3. Lunsford LD, Flickinger J, Lindner G, Maitz A. Stereotactic radiosurgery of the brain using the first United States 201 cobalt-60 source gamma knife. Neurosurgery. 1989;24(2):151–9.
4. Karikari IO, Isaacs RE. Minimally invasive transforaminal lumbar interbody fusion: a review of techniques and outcomes. Spine (Phila Pa). 1976;35(26 Suppl):S294–301.
5. Vaccaro AR, Chiba K, Heller JG, Patel T, Thalgott JS, Truumees E, Fischgrund JS, Craig MR, Berta SC, Wang JC. Bone grafting alternatives in spinal surgery. Spine J. 2002;2(3):206–15.
6. Leuthardt EC. What's holding us back? Understanding barriers to innovation in academic neurosurgery. Surg Neurol. 2006;66(4):347–9. discussion 349
7. Mayberg HS, Lozano AM, Voon V, McNeely HE, Seminowicz D, Hamani C, Schwalb JM, Kennedy SH. Deep brain stimulation for treatment-resistant depression. Neuron. 2005;45(5):651–60.

Chapter 4
Success in Academic Surgery: Innovation and Entrepreneurship Managing FDA Regulatory Requirements into a Positive Bridge for Commercial Success

Rita King and Russ King

Introduction: Clash of Medical Device Cultures

Surgeon entrepreneurs are uniquely powerful people. For those that I have known personally and professionally, the surgeon entrepreneur harnesses their passion as healers and deep need to create innovations that will help their patients. Their innovations have purpose, the power to change the future, and the promise to better medicine and patient outcomes. Furthermore, surgeon entrepreneurs tend to be prolific, and for these entrepreneurs one invention tends to lead to another. Many of the surgeon entrepreneurs I have spoken with have the conviction that their innovation will successfully enter the market and for the general measurable good of all. But there are many barriers that make successful entry into the US market with a medical innovation difficult. Moving an innovation from concept to point of care is frequently challenged by a lack of resources and money, a clearly defined market need, reimbursement issues, manufacturability issues, and successfully addressing the basic question "Is there a real business here and for who?"

Buried in the above challenges is the Food and Drug Administration (FDA). The FDA is a gate keeper for the US market when it comes to medical devices, biologics and drugs. Successfully commercializing a medical innovation means that the FDA agrees that the innovation is demonstrably safe in its intended use and demonstrably effective according to how it will be promoted. Demonstrating safety and efficacy means delivering evidence to the FDA according to rules, regulations, and established standards.

And there are a lot of rules, a lot of regulations, and a lot of standards.

R. King · R. King (✉)
MethodSense, Inc., Morrisville, NC, USA
e-mail: ritaking@methodsense.com; rking@methodsense.com

© Springer Nature Switzerland AG 2019
M. S. Cohen, L. Kao (eds.), *Success in Academic Surgery: Innovation and Entrepreneurship*, Success in Academic Surgery,
https://doi.org/10.1007/978-3-030-18613-5_4

Demonstrating safety and efficacy to the FDA requires close focus and attention to details (a lot of details), establishing and demonstrating you follow best practices, and the routinization of proven processes.

Every medical innovator knows they must "go through the FDA" and typically anticipates an uphill climb. Few though are prepared for the steep grade of the climb. For the surgeon entrepreneur, the effort to get through the FDA is usually more than just the work required together with the work's associated expenses. There is a deeper conflict physician innovators experience or should be prepared to experience when addressing FDA requirements.

The entrepreneur and innovator is driven by creativity and the desire to make a positive change in an agile environment. The FDA on the other hand is all about requirements, demonstration of claims in detail, and routinization. From this perspective, the innovator and the FDA are a poor match. One says fast, the other slow. One says agile, the other wants you to document fully and to the point of *ad nauseum*. One sees a clear line to better patient outcomes, while the other says "show me exactly how you have mitigated all the risks".

The catalogue of reactions we have seen to what the FDA requires of the physician innovator or entrepreneur ranges from sighs of frustration to outright vilification of the FDA. Nevertheless, the FDA is an unavoidable gatekeeper for medical innovation commercialization with a very important social and legal mission. Understanding the FDA and their needs, and thinking well in advance on how to integrate into entrepreneurial projects the demands of the FDA, is important for true medical device commercialization or at the very least mitigating some of the frustration associated with the process.

For nearly 20 years, our group at MethodSense, Inc. has worked with and helped entrepreneurs, emerging companies and well-established companies alike with regulatory issues and strategies. In what follows we offer some lessons learned about how entrepreneurs have successfully navigated the FDA. We focus on medical devices in large part because most innovation from the surgeon entrepreneur in our experience satisfies the legal definition of a medical device. There is a lot to say about medical devices and the FDA alone. Including biologics and pharmaceuticals as topics into the space available would be dilutive and more appropriate for other topics.

Our leadership at MethodSense collectively has 100 years of experience in regulated environments and we are still learning every single day. While this is an overview of the FDA process, it is NOT intended as regulatory advice about your particular circumstance or product. Instead, what follows is intended to be a high level story of lessons learned delivered in non-technical terms that will hopefully put you in a positive facing direction in preparation for future projects that must include the FDA.

The FDA Is Made of People

The Food and Drug Administration (the "FDA" or the "Agency") is a regulatory body. That is to say the FDA is a law enforcement agency. As a law enforcement agency, the FDA enforces for the most part what are called Administrative Laws that are designed to ensure product efficacy and public safety in the use of the products it oversees. According to the FDA website, the FDA enforces more than 200 laws and regulates more than $1 trillion worth of products.[1]

Other agencies you have heard of that enforce Administrative Laws include the Internal Revenue Service (IRS), Security Exchange Commission (SEC), and Immigration and Customs Enforcement (ICE). The Administrative Laws such agencies enforce can be found in the Code of Federal Regulations (CFR).[2] Examples of CFRs that the FDA enforces include (to name only a few):

- 21 PART 820 QUALITY SYSTEM REGULATION
- 21 CFR PART 807 ESTABLISHMENT REGISTRATION AND DEVICE LISTING FOR MANUFACTURERS AND INITIAL IMPORTERS OF DEVICES
- 21 CFR PART 11 ELECTRONIC RECORDS; ELECTRONIC SIGNATURES

The FDA's mandate includes a wide range of consumer health products including food, cosmetics, nutraceuticals, tobacco, biologics, pharmaceuticals, and medical devices. The FDA not only has oversight over these products that are produced domestically, but it also has oversight over the same products that are imported from non-domestic sources. The FDA is made up of a number of divisions devoted to these different product categories staffed by approximately 17,500 full time employees. The Center for Devices and Radiological Health (CDRH) is responsible for the regulation of medical devices and is staffed by more than 1,800 full time employees.[3]

The FDA enforces medical device laws through its product clearance or approval processes and inspections of manufacturers. As a law enforcement agency, the FDA can deny a product's entry into the market, as well as cite, fine, or prosecute companies or inventors for regulatory violations. While the FDA very seriously seeks to enforce regulations, they are equally serious as an organization and as individuals to see the quality of life and health of US citizens improve. The FDA is truly devoted to both the lawful use of medical devices as well as seeing the benefits of medical device innovation realized for those in need and as efficiently as possible.

This last point bears emphasis. After over 20 years working with the FDA, we have always been impressed by their devotion to benefiting the public. The laws, rules, and standards FDA personnel seek to develop and enforce are never capricious or arbitrary. Instead, they result from the hazards and harms the FDA has actually seen or ones they anticipate as part of the use of medical devices and from FDAs mission to protect those who are often the most vulnerable and in need of medical care.

According to the US Medical Device Industry Report, January 2018 by Bureau AWEX - New York, there are over 6500 medical device companies in the United

---

[1] See https://www.fda.gov/regulatoryinformation/lawsenforcedbyfda/default.htm

[2] See https://www.govinfo.gov/help/cfr

[3] See https://www.fda.gov/downloads/aboutfda/reportsmanualsforms/reports/budgetreports/ucm566335.pdf

States "valued at \$147.7 billion in 2016, and is expected to achieve even greater growth over the next few years, reaching a projected \$173 billion by 2019."[4] Additionally, medical devices continue to increase in complexity and the number of adverse events reporting on medical devices continues to rise dramatically.[5] Adding to this kind of pressure, the FDA is legally required to respond to product submission within certain timelines (e.g. 90 days for a 510(k)).

This all means that the FDA has a lot of ground to cover in fulfilling its mission in the face of limited resources. The FDA is commonly criticized for their job performance but we frequently find such criticism short sighted or myopic in the face of FDA's day to day challenges. This means that when it is time to communicate and work with the FDA, it will help your cause to do everything you can to make the FDA's job as easy as you can. The "Agency" is in the end made of people. If you build a working relationship with people in a manner that respects and helps them overcome their challenges, your working relationship will be more successful. And while you should not expect your FDA reviewer or inspector to be your friend, you can create with them success by understanding their challenges and helping them successfully meet their goals. In the end you will gain from the relationship.

The FDA Is Concerned about Products and Operations that Make Products

Innovators and entrepreneurs inexperienced with the FDA frequently have two misconceptions about the FDA when striking out in the arena of medical devices. First, they often conclude that they are not the legal manufacturer of a medical device. After all, they often argue, the device is manufactured by a contracted company who is actually building the product. Therefore, they often further conclude, the issues and burdens of regulatory compliance belong to the contracted company and not the innovator. Many times, contract manufacturing organizations (CMOs) will either reinforce this view or let it go unchallenged for the sake of securing business.

However, for the FDA a "Manufacturer means any legal person or entity engaged in the manufacture of a product subject to license under the act; "Manufacturer" also includes any legal person or entity who is an applicant for a license where the applicant assumes responsibility for compliance with the applicable product and establishment standards."[6] The key word here is "responsibility". Where the ultimate responsibility resides can most often be decided by the question "Where does

---

[4] See http://www.google.com/url?sa=t&rct=j&q=&esrc=s&source=web&cd=11&ved=2ahUKEw i2loWTsPDeAhWETt8KHcWZCkMQFjAKegQICRAC&url=http%3A%2F%2Fwww.awex-export.be%2Ffiles%2Flibrary%2FFiches-Pays%2FAMERIQUES%2FETATS-UNIS%2FThe-US-Medical-Device-Industry-2018.docx&usg=AOvVaw3vN-_HzP5-oPfwReOCbGSL

[5] See for example https://www.theexpertinstitute.com/medical-device-injuries-fda-data-reveals-increasing-risk/

[6] See https://www.accessdata.fda.gov/scripts/cdrh/cfdocs/cfCFR/CFRSearch.cfm?fr=600.3

the intellectual property reside and who enjoys the benefit of IP ownership? Is this with the contracted manufacturer? Or with the innovating company?" This does not mean that the contracted manufacturer has no responsibilities but it also means that unless the ownership of the device is relinquished to the contractor, the IP owner or the responsible party that can make final decisions about product designs and design changes bears ultimate responsibility for compliance as a legal manufacturer.

Second, innovators and entrepreneurs inexperienced with the FDA tend to devote their energies and resources around product development, prototyping, product improvements and regulatory concerns that directly impact the product. In many respects, this is very natural because the value of what they are creating is most often located in the product. However, FDA concerns extend well beyond the product to the operations that produce the product. The FDA wants assurances that the product that has been cleared or approved with its represented quality is the product that is manufactured…each and every time without exception. For this reason, the FDA (indeed all regulatory agencies globally) impose on companies Quality System Regulations or QSRs. In the FDA's case this is 21 CFR Part 820 QUALITY SYSTEM REGULATION or Good Manufacturing Practices (GMPs). In Europe and in general globally ISO 13485: 2016 Quality management systems -- Requirements for regulatory purposes is the QSR standard.

The commercialization of a medical device, therefore, can be said to have two regulatory components, a product component and company (or operational) component. The product component takes on for the most part the regulatory compliance of what you create while company component takes on the regulatory compliance of how you make what you create.

There is often no clear line between these two regulatory functions. Very often, however, the product component is referred to as "Regulatory Affairs" while the company component is typically referred to as "Quality Assurance." The work demands of these different roles usually necessitate separating the roles and distributing the work accordingly. But for startups we also see these functions consolidated to a single department, even a single individual, or farmed out to third party partners. Moreover, the work performed in the service of one role can very often impact the other. For example, the quality assurance task of creating a Risk Acceptance Policy and building a Risk Management File will always contribute to the Regulatory Affairs activity of creating a product pre-submission meeting package for FDA or be part of a product application for clearance or approval. Conversely, the Regulatory Affairs strategy for product clearance or approval can very quickly prioritize the activities of Quality Assurance activities.

In the end, the path of medical device commercialization must account for both the product and the company sides of the regulatory equation. Ignoring or delaying inappropriately the company part, i.e. the Quality Assurance part, of what it means to commercialize a medical device invariably in our experience creates risks and costs that are otherwise avoidable. Medical device companies need as a matter of law at the time of product clearance or approval a fully compliant Quality Management System (QMS). After product clearance or approval all medical device companies are open to FDA inspection for compliance monitoring purposes.

Delaying the development of your quality program and QMS creates additional expense and potential mistakes from a hurried and harried exercise of formalizing processes. Further, records that reflect following those processes may require retrospective management and creation from emails, documents, napkins, etc., which likewise has a tendency to result in mistakes observable during FDA inspection. There are strategies and tactics to develop your Quality Assurance program and QMS in a manner that tracks the regulatory maturation of your product (which we will mention further below).

FDA Medical Device Commercialization Paths

The FDA utilizes a risk-based approach when licensing medical devices for the US market. The FDA segments devices into three risk classifications, Class I, Class II and Class III where Class I products are the least risky and Class III the most risky (see Table below). The higher the risk, the higher the evidentiary threshold for demonstrating product safety and efficacy.

Class I examples: stethoscopes, bandages, wheelchairs	Class II examples: ultrasonic diagnostic equipment, x-rays, needles	Class III examples: balloon catheters, pacemakers, heart valves
• Low risk devices that are simple in design • Self-register product with the FDA • Most are exempt from pre-market requirements • QMS normally comply with 21 CFR Part 820 General Controls, though some devices are exempt	• Medium risk devices that are more complex in design • 510(k) pre-market approval process is required for most • QMS must comply with 21 CFR Part 820: Special Controls (Design Controls)	• High risk devices • FDA shall inspect facility • QMS must comply with 21 CFR Part 820 • Clinical trials likely • Malfunction is absolutely unacceptable

A great portion of a device commercialization strategy's cost and time-to-market is determined by the product's risk classification. That is, a Class II product has a significantly easier path to market than a Class III product, and a Class I product has the easiest path to market.

Class I products require Establishment Registration and Medical Device Listing[7] as well as compliance to FDA Quality System General Controls. This low bar for

---

[7] See https://www.fda.gov/medicaldevices/deviceregulationandguidance/howtomarketyourdevice/registrationandlisting/default.htm

medical device market entry is rarely something we see as a medical device consulting firm for the simple reason that products falling under this category are typically very simple or commodities and do not require any specialized knowledge for navigating the FDA.

Of these three risk classifications, the most frequently used FDA process we encounter is the pre-market notification or 510(k) process. Medium risk Class II devices have in general (and at a very high level) the potential for a greater medical impact on patient care than Class I products. More importantly, a Class II medical device represents a more attractive investment opportunity than other more difficult regulatory paths because receiving the 510(k) and consequently the freedom to market the product and produce revenues can happen for fewer dollars and in less time. Consequently, entrepreneurs looking for capital will have a wider investor audience that will have an interest in their company than for products that require De Novo or a PMA.

510(k) Clearance

The 510(k) process is designed to demonstrate that a new medical device is as safe and effective as a device that has already been cleared by the FDA. This means that instead of proving safety and efficacy via clinical trials, you demonstrate safety and efficacy by showing a Class II device is *substantially equivalent* to a predicate device that has already been shown to be safe and effective.

So, what exactly is substantial equivalence? A device is substantially equivalent if, in comparison to a predicate, it has:

- The same intended use as the predicate; and
- The same technological characteristics as the predicate;

   OR

- The same intended use as the predicate; and
- Has different technological characteristics and the information submitted to FDA:

   - Does not raise new questions of safety and effectiveness; and
   - Demonstrates that the device is at least as safe and as effective as the legally marketed device

Developing a 510(k) submission involves developing a formal argument that establishes for your product substantial equivalence to the predicate. In the course of developing the submission, you will do what the predicate device did for product clearance. If the predicate device was cleared just using performance data demonstrating safety and efficacy, then so will you. If the predicate device established safety through IEC 60601-1 rather than IEC 61010, then so will you. If the predicate used clinical data for product clearance, then so must you. Therefore, the chosen predicate device will play an important role in determining the time and cost to market.

From a business and strategy perspective, it is important to realize that there is a dynamic between the intended use or indications for use as an FDA cleared or approved medical device and how you can promote the medical device. For example, if an in vitro diagnostic (IVD) is cleared to detect a particular biomarker associated with cancer, then that does not mean you can claim that the IVD diagnoses cancer. It means that you can claim that the IVD detects a particular biomarker and that's all. Promoting or selling a medical device for something other than for that which it was approved is illegal. The FDA refers to such products as "adulterated".

But entrepreneurs should view the relationship between a product's intended use and the business goals of their company prior to approval in a much more nuanced way. Many surgeon entrepreneurs are creating medical devices that are genuine platforms and designed to fulfill multiple clinical purposes or address multiple different statements of use. Other medical devices have a versatility or as an invention the clinical power to address more than one discrete medical condition, each of which might be captured by a different statement of intended use. In such cases, it is not uncommon in our medical device consulting practice to have to make a choice about the intended use of a product and address questions like: Which intended use should we use to pursue product clearance? The intended use that makes for an easier 510(k)? The intended use that goes after a larger potential market? The intended use that creates for competitors the greatest barrier for market entry?

These kind of choices make for an opportunity because it gives you the option to align with a regulatory strategy such factors such as:

- The scope of work to time to market,
- Indication of use to target market,
- Business plan to capital resource
- Runway to business goals

The bottom line is that your regulatory strategy is more than just something that is "nice to have" but rather should be a strategic contribution to your business plans.

Non-traditional 510(k) or De Novo

Sometimes, you may find yourself in a situation where your device has no substantially equivalent predicate. Or you may file a traditional 510(k) application and the FDA rejects the application with a Non-Substantially Equivalent designation. If either is the case, you may still have a Class II pathway in the De Novo application process.

The FDA automatically designates a medical device that does not have a predicate as a Class III device. Prior to 2012, the avenues for medical device innovators whose products had no predicate were forced down the burdensome PMA pathway even though many understood that the risk profile of their product did not rise to the risk profile level of Class III devices. Inventors placed in this situation often argued that: "I agree that my medical device might be harmful if things go wrong. But the injuries are always minor if they occur at all and permanent injury or death will never occur. It's nonsense to categorize my device as a Class III device." In 2012 the FDA responded to this circumstance with the creation of the De Novo pathway.

If you can clearly demonstrate that the risk profile of your predicateless medical device does not rise above the risk profile of a Class I or Class II device, then the De Novo path to clearance as a Class II product may be available to you.[8] The De Novo process requires a pre-submission meeting with and permission from the FDA to follow the De Novo process. Though De Novo very often represents a less expensive and more efficient route to market than a Pre-Market Approval or PMA pathway for Class III devices, the De Novo process will be more arduous than the traditional 510(k) because it will likely require clinical studies and the De Novo process itself can add 6–18 months in FDA review time to the normal 510(k) clearance process.

There are a number of things you can look out for if considering De Novo. The De Novo application will require clinical data to support safety and efficacy. If a difficult and expensive clinical trial is needed, then there may be little to no cost or efficiency difference between the De Novo and filing a PMA. Also, the pre-submission De Novo meeting should seek to address as much as the time allotted by the FDA will allow. In additional to your risk based arguments for why you qualify for De Novo, you will ideally want to present your clinical protocol and perhaps additional questions in order to resolve potential regulatory vulnerabilities. Also remember that once your De Novo application is cleared by the FDA, other medical device companies competing with yours can use your cleared Class II product as a predict device for filing a traditional 510(k). So your successful completion of the more difficult De Novo path can make your competitor's life much easier.

Pre-Market Approval or PMA

Class III high risk medical devices require FDA Pre-market approval or a PMA.[9] A PMA is the most difficult regulatory pathway, requiring more money and time, for medical device commercialization. Josh Makower of Stanford University famously reported in the 2010 report "FDA Impact on U.S. Medical Technology Innovation" that the average cost to take a 510(k) product from concept to market is $31 million, and that roughly 77% of that amount is spent on tasks related to FDA regulation. High-risk PMA costs averaged $94 million, the report states, with $75 million of that spent on "stages linked to the FDA." While in the experience of our medical device consulting practice these costs descriptions are 'hyperbolic', the relative

---

[8] See FDA Guidance De Novo Classification Process (Evaluation of Automatic Class III Designation)

[9] See https://www.fda.gov/medicaldevices/deviceregulationandguidance/howtomarketyourdevice/premarketsubmissions/premarketapprovalpma/

difference between a 510(k) and a PMA is noteworthy: PMAs are significantly more costly than a 510(k).

The cost associated with a PMA is generally associated with the higher regulatory expectation for quality and the likelihood that you will need clinical trials for product approval. Manufacturers must meet FDA quality inspector's expectations prior to receiving a PMA and very often high risk devices such as heart valves and pacemakers pose interesting and generally expensive challenges for successful clinical trials. Since they are high risk devices, the FDA will likely treat Class III medical devices as Significant Risk devices and require an Investigational Device Exemption before allowing clinical trials to move forward. And the rigor required for a PMA goes on.

From a business perspective, many potential investors get skittish around Class III products. Angles and Angel Groups tend to avoid them because the amount of money required, the risks associated with, and the time to market for such projects. Institutional investors who are willing to take the long view on cost and time to market will reflect these risks in their term sheets.

On the other hand, not many have the right resources to pursue a PMA. If you successfully receive a PMA, the PMA as a path to market becomes its own barrier to potential competition. Moreover, the right personnel or consulting assistance familiar with the demands of a PMA can convert what is otherwise a "scary project" into a successful project.

Combination Products

Combination products are FDA regulated products that incorporate a medical device component with a drug or biologic component.[10] Examples of combination products include automated and manual prefilled syringes, contract agent injectors, and drug-eluting stents. The medical device component of a combination product may have the sole purpose of delivering a drug or biologic such as a syringe or the medical device component may provide an additional purpose as in the case of the drug-eluting stent.

Combination products pose extra regulatory complexities because they incorporate products that by themselves would fall under different product regulations. Typically the review process for a combination will include FDA regulatory authorities from the CDRH or the Drug (CDER) and /or Biologics (CBER) divisions of the FDA as appropriate.

Of particular interest to the innovator entrepreneur and a product's investors is which FDA division will take the lead (or have primary jurisdiction) on a combination product project under the belief that, for example, if CDRH takes the lead, the project will be easier. This may be a false hope, however, because in our experience each division gets their say and can advance or trump regulatory submissions regardless of who takes the lead.

---

[10] See https://www.fda.gov/CombinationProducts/AboutCombinationProducts/ucm118332.htm

The FDA acknowledges the complexities of combination products and through the FDA Office of Combination Products[11] works to help both the FDA and combination product companies understand and effectively deal with these complexities.

IVDs and LTDs

In-vitro Diagnostics (IVDs) are medical devices designed for the in-vitro examination of specimens derived from the human body solely or principally to provide information for diagnostic, monitoring or compatibility purposes. IVDs will include an assay and the means to deliver information about the assay. The information delivery could be part of the assay itself (e.g. a paper strip), or come from a reader provided by a third party, or the assay developer may create their own proprietary reader. Most IVD entrepreneurs are faced with making two different kind of choices:

1. What will the IVD do?

    (a) Will it diagnose? or
    (b) Will it provide information to the health care professional who will diagnose?

2. How will I take the IVD to market?

    (a) As a medical device?
    (b) As a Laboratory Developed Test?

The FDA assumes that IVDs that diagnose (e.g. positively identifies that at patient has cancer) as a Class III device unless you can effectively argue that it is a Class II device. Companion diagnostics, or IVDs that help assess the effectiveness of pharmaceutical or biologic therapy, likewise tend to be considered Class III devices by the FDA unless they are convinced otherwise.

More frequently, IVD developers seek to introduce an IVD as an adjunct to current standards of care, providing information to the clinician that helps them form a diagnosis. This typically gives the IVD a Class II risk classification where the regulatory path to market is typically a 510(k) or De Novo.

IVD entrepreneurs who find themselves with a device that has the capability or promise of diagnosing will very often initially take the IVD through the FDA in a 510(k) as an adjunctive device for the sake of an initial shorter path to market. Subsequently, once revenues are realized they will return to developing claims for diagnosing in a subsequent FDA submission. This kind of approach can make a business plan around and IVD more attractive to investors.

Laboratory Developed Tests (LDTs) are also diagnostics that perform in-vitro examinations of specimens from the human body. The FDA defines LDTs as medical

---

[11] See https://www.fda.gov/aboutfda/centersoffices/officeofmedicalproductsandtobacco/officeofscienceandhealthcoordination/ucm2018184.htm

devices that are designed and manufactured in a single laboratory. The history between the FDA and LDTs, and in particular their more recent history, is rather complicated and perhaps best told by the FDA itself (see the FDA website Laboratory Developed Tests[12]). The short history of it is that as LDTs began to emerge they were relatively simple and posed minimal risks to patients and users. Though the FDA viewed LDTs as medical devices, they applied to LDTs what is called "enforcement discretion" as a way to balance the benefits they deliver in the face of their low risk. Enforcement discretion means that the FDA chooses not to enforce medical device regulations for LDTs though they reserve the right to reverse their position at some later time.

As LDTs have become increasingly complex the FDA has become concerned about the concomitant increasing risks associated with LDTs. In 2014 the FDA responded by proposing to abandon enforcement discretion and regulate LDTs.[13] The laboratory test industry, a critical component to health care and a significant industry on its own, protested loudly causing an FDA retreat from its plans for at least the present time.

The FDA position of enforcement discretion creates a potential opportunity for entrepreneurs who seek a commercialization path for their diagnostic yet want to avoid FDA regulations and expectations for clearance or approval. This pathway typically includes either the entrepreneur starting a laboratory for running their diagnostic tests or licensing their technology to an established laboratory for them to develop the LDT.

But the LDT route is not without regulatory burdens. In order for a LDT to be reimbursed, the laboratory in which the test takes place must be Clinical Laboratory Improvement Amendments (CLIA) certified unless you can obtain a CLIA Waiver (typically awarded to very simple tests). CLIA is enforced by the Centers for Medicare and Medicaid Services (CMS) who also reimburse companies for these tests. The demands for CLIA certification requirements are generally:

- Compliance with relevant federal, state and local laboratory laws
- Request and document patient info/specimen info as appropriate
- Document procedures and procedure changes
- Verify and maintain documentation regarding a test's performance is similar to the manufacturer's claims for accuracy, precision and reportable range
- Perform calibration and calibration verification as outlined in the manufacturer's instructions or at least every 6 months and checked at a minimum three levels that are within the reportable range of the test.

---

[12] See https://www.fda.gov/MedicalDevices/ProductsandMedicalProcedures/InVitroDiagnostics/LaboratoryDevelopedTests/default.htm

[13] See FDA, Draft Guidance for Industry, FDA Staff, and Clinical Laboratories: FDA Notification and Medical Device Reporting for Laboratory Developed Tests (LDTs) (Oct. 3, 2014); FDA, Draft Guidance for Industry, Framework for Regulatory Oversight of Laboratory Developed Tests (LDTs) (Oct. 3, 2014).

- Employ qualified Lab directors
- Follow an appropriate performing Quality Control (QC) plan
- Follow a Record and Specimen Retention Plan
- Assess quality throughout the total testing process.

Starting a LDT company from a university or hospital system environment has a reputation for being a limited business opportunity. Endorsement to use an LDT from the local friendly environment can encourage and excite the entrepreneur about an opportunity; but expanding the subscription base of an LTD service to a broader audience outside the entrepreneur's immediate ecosystem tends to be very difficult.

Alternatively, laboratory companies or organizations are typically interested in licensing an LDT technology if the LDT fits into their current portfolio of testing services, is part of a platform where testing services can be expanded, and the LDT satisfies a need for which the laboratory does not have to create a market. So a lot of stars must cross to successfully license an LTD to a laboratory. Moreover, the regulatory story on LDTs has not ended because FDA may still transition away from enforcement discretion.

When Should You Talk to the FDA?

All conversations with the FDA are good to have. Not all conversations with the FDA are useful for product commercialization.

We commonly hear from medical device developers, particularly for first time entrepreneurs out of academic settings, that they "had a great conversation with the FDA." Frequently these conversations take place at meetings or conferences the FDA hosted or attended. Often, entrepreneurs take the words they hear from the FDA as a sign about the commercial value of their product, as an indication of the regulatory pathway of their product, or the ease or difficulty of that regulatory pathway. And such communications and advice should be taken just as seriously as the valuable input one may receive from any other experienced medical device professional. But the most important words you will hear will be from the FDA team who can clear or approve the product for the market, i.e. the reviewers of your application. In the end, what the FDA Directory of Regulatory Science, or the Deputy Director for Science and Strategic Initiatives, or Director of Knowledge Management, or etc., is not as important as the reviewer(s) recommendations regarding product license. So the question about when to begin talking to the FDA and how to speak effectively with the FDA for the purposes of commercialization is an important one.

A common (and very simplistic) graphic that describes a successful commercialization path for a medical device can look like this:

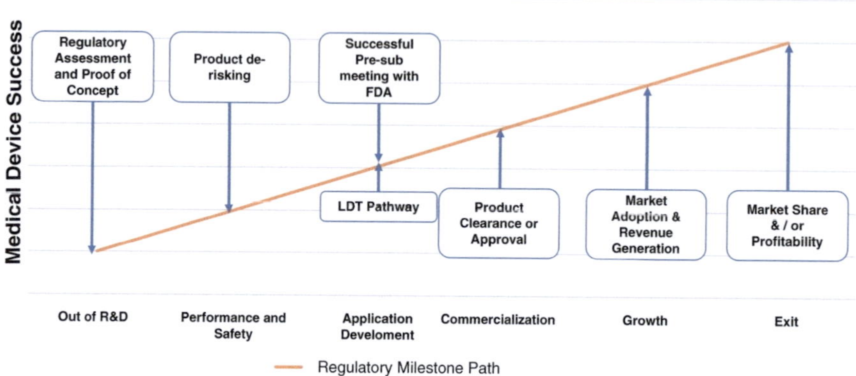

The best time to talk to the FDA for the sake of moving a medical technology successfully through commercialization occurs at a certain point of product maturity so that you can get to a desired end point in the discussion. Discussions with the FDA based on a product or product information that is too immature for the discussion can easily result in FDA feedback that reflects the immaturity of the information presented which can take you down a misguided path and create unnecessary risks and costs. The FDA always reserves the right to say, "Yes, at that time I thought one way about your product, but now that I am better informed I think differently." Reducing the risk of delays and backtracking over expensive ground, such as having to refile an application as a De Novo rather than a 510(k) or redoing clinical studies so that the FDA can have confidence in a products safety or efficacy, is critical.

Product or product information maturity in the way we are thinking here is much more than a robust prototype. It means thinking about and preparing product information in a manner that adequately informs the FDA about the product and anticipates relevant FDA concerns and questions so that conversations can move in a direction that benefits you. Product preparations in this regard should include a justified understanding of the regulatory status of the product and the right information about your device that enables the FDA to answer critical question in a manner you can count on for making important commercialization decisions. There is no rule we can cite for when the right regulatory understanding, sufficient information, and critical questions converge except to say that experience will tell us when we are ready. But we can describe how to establish your regulatory understanding and best practices for developing the information you will need.

Regulatory Roadmaps

A good Regulatory Roadmap will establish your regulatory strategy by identifying whether your device is a Class I, II, or III device as well as the three letter Product Code associated with your product.[14] It should identify all the major milestones for product clearance or approval including safety testing, biocompatibility testing, clinical data needs, the Quality Management System requirements you will need to meet, and the regulations the Quality System must satisfy. Most importantly, the Regulatory Roadmap will provide justificatory arguments for its conclusion, not just opinions. This means the Roadmap will justify the 510(k) pathway with a preliminary yet evidentiary argument for a particular predicate device. Alternatively, the Roadmap may justify the De Novo pathway with an argument for why the risk profile does not exceed a Class II risk classification. Or, finally, the Roadmap may justify the PMA pathway with an argument about why the risk profile in fact exceeds a Class II risk classification.

A Regulatory Roadmap grounded in justified arguments gives you a number of advantages. It can serve as a basis for product and business milestone identification and planning including the type of discussion you would benefit most with the FDA in your commercialization journey. Your Regulatory Roadmap should further tell you the milestones you should budget for and enable you to present potential investors in a confident manner with product commercialization requirements.

Knowing your Device: Design Controls and Risk Assessments

The FDA (and medical device regulators global) takes a risk management approach to the industry. This means that their focus is prioritized by risk when it comes to developing QSRs, inspections, and the development of new regulations and guidance.

We discussed earlier how FDA product clearance or approval carries with it the expectation that you will comply with QSRs. For medical device companies, this typically means at least compliance with 21 CFR Part 820, also known as Good Manufacturing Practices (GMPs). GMPs take a risk management approach to the manufacture of medical devices and forces device expertise. GMPs in general:

- Are an FDA-mandated system of product design
- Require you to document the evolution of the life of your product
- Apply a market-first product development focus
- Require a team-oriented approach to product commercialization
- As a process, tend to challenge product design to the point of improvement

21 CFR Part 820 prescribes specific design controls, or processes, that occurs in phases which when followed move a product along a commercialization path and are often characterized in the following way:

- Design and Development Planning
- Design and Development Input/Output

---

[14] For FDA information about product codes see https://www.fda.gov/MedicalDevices/ DeviceRegulationandGuidance/Overview/ClassifyYourDevice/ucm051637.htm

- Design and Development Verification
- Design Validation
- Design Transfer
- Design Changes
- Design History File

Design controls should work as a risk prevention approach to the quality of your medical device. Risk prevention is an efficient and cost-effective way to control manufacturing processes and maintain quality. While it may not be possible to eliminate all potential risks, we consistently observe in our clients a very poor appetite for realized risk that was otherwise avoidable. Design controls often include:

- Establishing intended use and design inputs
- A design plan
- Periodic design reviews throughout the design process
- Confirmation that the design outputs conform to the design inputs through design verification ("Are we making the device according to the design?")
- Design validation ("Are we making the right device?")
- Translation of the design into manufacturable specifications
- Clear documentation of the entire process in a design history file or DHF

If implemented early and well, design controls create a number of surprisingly valuable results including:

- a better-documented product that is more attractive to acquire or license,
- a more efficient development cycle due to a reduction of mistakes thanks to early analysis of key questions about the medical device itself
- a very practical way to develop early on best practices that are necessary for a medical device company

Product risk assessments are part of the design process and play a particularly important role in the early stages of a product leading up to your first formal FDA communication. Your Quality Management System will include a Risk Policy or Standard Operating Procedure (SOP) and a Risk Acceptance Criteria. The purpose of a product risk assessment is to demonstrate that you fully understand the risks associated with your product and you understand the mitigating steps that need to be in place to ensure a safe product.

When developing a risk assessment, you will first identify all the hazards and harms that may be realized in the use and operation of your device. After hazards and harms are identified, the application of the Risk Policy and Risk Acceptance Criteria results in the identification of risks, together with their severity and depending on your risk policy their expected frequency. The next step is to identify the controls that will be put in place to prevent realizing those risks. Controls may include how the device inherently works, labeling to mitigate inappropriate use of the product, or how it is manufactured. Once the controls are identified, you then address any remaining residual risks associated with the device including any residual risks that might be generated by the controls themselves.

Many product innovators and beginner medical device entrepreneurs we help sometimes resist product risk assessments either because they (wishfully) believe there are no risks associated with their products, or if shown the light of day, product risks will make the product less desirable or important. Neither is the case. The FDA will typically require a risk assessment for your pre-submission meeting and as part of the product submission. Moreover, risk assessments are a very natural complement to a product's science where the goal is a particular kind of knowledge, in this case knowledge about how the medical device might actually work and behave in the market for which it is intended.

There are other ways the entrepreneur and emerging company can better understand their medical device. They may for example perform a predicate analysis if they are filing a 510(k), bench testing, preliminary electrical performance testing with a test lab, conduct animal studies, or assessing the manufacturability of their device to acquire some basic knowledge about their product that may impact the outcome of a discussion with the FDA about their products commercialization.

Meeting with the FDA

Formal discussions with the FDA that directly impact the commercialization of a medical device are broadly referred to as Q-Submissions (Q-Subs) and include what are also known as Pre-Submission (Pre-Sub) meetings. Q-Subs have various purposes that may include:

- Informational Meetings
- Study Risk Determination
- Formal Early Collaboration Meetings
- Submission Issue Meeting
- Day 100 Meeting for PMA Applications
- Pre-Submission Meetings

Most of the Q-Subs we see medical device companies request are pre-subs. The reasons for a scheduling a pre-pub is to obtain FDA feedback to important questions prior to an intended application, questions that might include:

- How the FDA might apply regulations to a novel technology
- How to manage "first of a kind" indication or a new indication for an existing device
- Clarification from the FDA about the regulatory strategy of a device when the device does not clearly fall in an established regulatory pathway
- Gaining FDA guidance on specific issues related to nonclinical and/or preclinical study protocols, before initiating the studies

Pre-subs with the FDA represent an incredible opportunity to clearly understand Agency expectations for successful product clearance or approval. Pre-subs also represent a genuine opportunity to establish a positive relationship with reviewers, get them excited about your innovation, and establish in them confidence that you are going to do the right thing by complying with regulations.

The following kind of scenario can help clarify when a pre-sub might be desirable and how it might proceed:

> An emerging company concludes that its medical device should follow a 510(k) regulatory pathway but the company also recognizes the potential that the FDA may disagree because there are important technological differences between the company's product and the candidate predicate device. The company has staked a lot on a 510(k) regulatory strategy with the development of budgets, timelines and representations to investors. Confirming with the FDA that the identified 510(k) strategy will be accepted will help the business move forward.

Addressing this scenario will generally mean formally requesting a pre-sub meeting for which the company will prepare a pre-sub package for FDA review. The Pre-Sub package will include technical and risk information about the product and the questions you want the FDA to address. In this case, the Pre-Sub package may include a predicate analysis comparing in detail the similarities and differences between your product and the candidate predicate, developing a risk assessment that demonstrates that the risk posed by the technical differences of your product does not create additional risks when compared to the predicate, and a conclusion that your product qualifies for the 510(K) process. The Pre-Sub will ask the FDA "Do you agree that the product qualifies for the 510(k) process?" and perhaps other critical questions answers to which will help you move forward successfully.

The FDA will review the Pre-Sub package and 70 days after the meeting date agreed to and respond to the package 5 days (or so) prior to the scheduled meeting with feedback that will likely be the focus of the meeting. The meeting can take place by phone conference call or in person at the FDA and the meeting will last 1 h during which the FDA will provide the feedback to the questions asked. After the meeting, the company submitting the package will author and submit to the FDA pre-sub meeting minutes which the FDA will accept or amend.

Depending on the complexity of your device and the regulatory issues associated with your device, you may find a need for more than one pre-sub or Q-sub meeting. In our practice we have seen the need for up to seven pre-sub where the issues involved were difficult for the medical device company and FDA reviewers alike. Once the communication around a pre-sub submission is underway, particularly after the initial pre-sub meeting, there are occasions when "picking up the phone" is possible with an assigned reviewer with questions that do not require the participation of multiple FDA reviewers.

There is no doubt that preparing for a pre-sub takes time and can create up-front costs. But whatever is created in the service of a pre-sub meeting should be usable down the road in your submissions and you get the added benefit of answering critical questions in a manner that can prevent future mistakes and the need to go back and redo work you may have thought was completed. But with a stable product, your regulatory path defined and your critical questions answered, what remains is the work required to complete the requirements of a submission in a manner that meets the expectations of the FDA.

Question Shortcuts

Investor expectations and demands, limited resources and short business runways, the natural impatience of the innovator anxious to improve the lives and health of patients, and other pressures often have entrepreneurs struggling to make the ends meet. Often we see medical device entrepreneurs beginning complex projects and starting companies with a view toward prudent fiscal and operational management of the project. As the pressures grow, prudence can evolve into taking shortcuts in the form of skipping steps along the way and completing steps in a less robust way than you might have completed them with fewer pressures.

It is worth being very wary of shortcuts. Accelerating the achievement of certain regulatory steps is one thing, but hastening the completion of a milestone by skipping steps or elevating the work to a high level in lieu of the detail needed to fully achieve a regulatory milestone always in our experience creates the long way around and ultimately becomes more costly.

It is not uncommon to hear from a medical device company under pressure an argument that takes the following form: "The FDA wants us to do X. We know that doing X will cost us $Y. We really cannot afford $Y right now, so let's try to justify not doing X for the sake of saving $Y."

On numerous occasions we have seen companies take this path and usually with a poor outcome. First, while it is true that FDA personnel in general have limited experience in business environments, they are still very smart, are scientifically astute, know the purpose of the regulations inside and out, and have seen more than their share of the wordsmithing and dodges. If the FDA says they need something, then they need it or its equivalent. In every scenario we have seen like the one describe above, the cost of attempting to avoid a defined need of the FDA has always resulted in increased costs and lost time. In short, be very wary about "shortcuts" and make certain that when you choose to take a shortcut that you are truly accelerating your business and not jeopardizing an FDA need required for your business' success.

Post Product Clearance or Approval

What happens after product clearance or approval? Frankly, the hard part which includes operating your business as prescribed by your Quality Management System and remaining auditable in anticipation of an FDA inspection, executing on your sales and marketing plan, growing your market share and revenues, staying competitive in the face of companies who try to take away your customers, and achieving the business expectations of investors looking for an exit. While meeting the expectations of the FDA is necessary, it is arguably not the most difficult milestone of an emerging business.

Very often post product clearance is hard on the innovator entrepreneur in other ways. Investors and with their expectations will typically assume that achieving the exit they are after will require an executive whose experience includes accelerating a business to an exit. If the founder of a company with investors does not have this experience, the investors may want to put in place an executive that does have such experience for the sake of protecting their investment. This may mean that the founder entrepreneur is moved from CEO or President to some other position or removed altogether depending on the founder's relationship with investors and the company's Board of Directors. But the disappointment and hard feelings this might create can be manage by the founder anticipating it.

Some Last Thoughts

In summary creating a thoughtful regulatory roadmap with a process in place to complete each step along the path will save a company both time, money, and in many cases frustration related to getting their product to market. While the FDA has many rules and regulations to keep the consumer safe while using new technologies, they are an important group to engage and work with through this often complex process. While regulations for devices, drugs, and diagnostics have a clear path, regulations around digital health products and Artificial Intelligence are still being navigated as more and more of these technologies are being created. The entrepreneur has many options and potential roads to market, so time spent focusing on the correct regulatory roadmap is time well spent and will provide the best chance for commercial success!

Chapter 5
Getting Funding for a Surgical Innovation: Opportunities and Challenges

Reda Jaber

Introduction

With change comes opportunity and there has never been a more opportune time than now for an academic surgeon to capitalize on a vast and diverse funding landscape in their effort to bridge the gap between research and commercialization.

As the healthcare industry continues to transform in dramatic ways, surgeons with groundbreaking contributions spanning virtually all areas of innovation—from medical devices, drugs, health IT, and other emerging technologies—now stand on the brink of enormous possibility.

Unquestionably, the "Golden Age of Medpreneurship" is in full swing with increasing access to capital, declining cost of technology, and the world's information instantly available with a simple Google or PubMed search. This means more medical entrepreneurs than ever before now have the resources in-hand to forge new startups with dramatic market potential at an unrivaled pace.

While the funding landscape and existing market continue to rapidly evolve, the concept of "surgeon as inventor" is one with historical legitimacy. In fact, one needs to look no further than Dr. William Halsted—the "Father of Modern Surgery"—as a prime example. Halsted, who practiced at the turn of the century, not only contributed largely to the founding of modern anesthesiology, but pioneered several types of surgical procedures. He also introduced rubber surgical gloves into the operating room through an industry collaboration with the Goodyear Rubber Company in 1890. Halsted's career epitomized the concept of a surgeon able to translate his daily expertise into vital and tangible medical advancements.

R. Jaber (⊠)
IncWell, Birmingham, MI, USA
e-mail: reda@theincwell.net

© Springer Nature Switzerland AG 2019
M. S. Cohen, L. Kao (eds.), *Success in Academic Surgery: Innovation and Entrepreneurship*, Success in Academic Surgery,
https://doi.org/10.1007/978-3-030-18613-5_5

Although circumstances have clearly changed dramatically since Halsted's era, the collision of interwoven factors in today's healthcare market have made it ripe for disruption by new players and models. Such factors include:

- U.S. healthcare spending reached $3.5 trillion in 2017 and is projected to reach nearly $6 trillion by 2026 according to CMS. Notably, an estimated 40% of the $3.5 trillion industry could have been circumvented with more efficient products and models, according to industry sources.
- Nearly 20 million people have gained health insurance since 2010 as a result of comprehensive health care reform (Affordable Care Act). This influx of new patients with substantially improved access to care necessitates a more efficient and cost-effective delivery model.
- A mandate requiring electronic medical records (EMR) utilization has contributed to a Big Data revolution in healthcare.
- People are living longer: 10,000 baby boomers are reaching age 65 every day. This demographic will increasingly utilize more healthcare products and services as they age.
- Millennials are also changing the healthcare industry. Nicknamed "The Now Generation," these consumers value convenience, connectivity, and transparency in healthcare more than previous generations.
- Technology in general is evolving with emerging technologies and trends such as sensor miniaturization, telemedicine, artificial intelligence, internet of medical things (IoMT), blockchain for healthcare, and augmented or virtual reality.

The Investor Mindset

Startup investments are inherently risky and generally the goal is to both de-risk the business at each stage of funding and create value. "Early-stage" investors, including angel investors and early-stage VC funds, are more risk-tolerant, while "late-stage" investors, including late-stage VC funds and private equity funds, are more risk-averse. Early-stage investors are willing to take on the inherent risk at earlier stages because there is potential for a higher reward.

When investors consider a startup for funding, their goal is to evaluate both the upside potential and downside risk associated with the company, including the following themes:

- **The Value Proposition:** Is it possible the company will create value for a significant number of people/organizations? Is it a unique and superior solution to a significant obstacle?
- **The Market:** How significant is the market opportunity for the proposed product or service? Is the company in a growing industry?
- **The Leadership Team:** Is the team qualified to run the venture?

- **Scale:** Is it possible the company will achieve significant growth and earn significant revenue in the next 5 years?
- **The Ask:** Is the company asking for the right amount of money to meet significant growth milestones? Is the company's planned use of funds appropriate?

Investors will also want to understand how the entrepreneur plans to manage the following risks:

- **Technical Risk:** Does the product or process actually work?
- **Financial Risk:** Can the company raise enough money to achieve the next milestone?
- **Regulatory Risk:** Can the company get through the FDA regulatory approval process?
- **Intellectual Property Risk:** Is the company infringing on anyone's patents and is it protecting its innovation properly so that no one can infringe on its patent?
- **Market Risk:** Will there be enough demand for the product by the time it gets to market?

Funding Rounds Explained

Very few entrepreneurs are able to fully "bootstrap" a company without external capital—especially in the healthcare space where large amounts of funding are generally required to get medical technologies to market. A typical startup goes through several rounds of funding to achieve the appropriate milestones, which can include FDA regulatory approval, commercialization, profitability, and eventually a liquidation event for the shareholders. As startups advance beyond the grant stage—the funding levels, company valuation and expectations from investors naturally increase (Table 5.1).

Grant Stage

Non-dilutive government- or foundation-sponsored grants that can support key research for the company, or academic funding meant to support faculty development, are often the first sources of funding for new surgical innovations. Grants provide support to innovators at a key time when the technology may be perceived as "too risky" or "unproven" by traditional investors. Therefore, these funds are often used to build a body of research publications that establish a preclinical or technical proof of concept. This stage is a key time for a company to build its core intellectual property, which can be a cornerstone of value for the company in future rounds.

Table 5.1 Startup funding rounds

	Grant Stage	Pre-Seed/Seed	Series A	Series B+	IPO
Typical funding amount	Variable	<$1 million	$1–10 million	$10–30 million	>$30 million
Typical company valuation	N/A (non-dilutive)	$1–6 million	$5–20 million	$30–140 million	>$150 million
Common investors	• Government-Sponsored Grants (ex. NIH, DARPA, SBIR) • Academic Institutions • Foundations/Non-Profits	• Friends & Family • Angels • Family Offices • Accelerators • Early-Stage Venture Capital	• Angels • Family Offices • Venture Capital	• Late-stage Venture Capital • Corporate Venture • Private Equity • Hedge Funds	• Corporate Venture • Hedge Funds • Investment Banks

Pre-Seed/Seed

Pre-seed and seed rounds are considered to be the very first form of funding open to startups beyond the grant stage. These funds are often used by the company to make key hires, develop a prototype, quantify market readiness, and run key experiments.

For companies with lower regulatory hurdles (for example, Health IT or Class I Medical Devices), the ultimate goal of this round may be to get to market and start generating revenue. Health IT companies will focus on software development, and Class I Medical Device companies will focus on product development and manufacturing.

For companies with higher regulatory hurdles (Class II/III Medical Devices, pharmaceuticals), these rounds attempt to address the so-called "translational funding gap" which often lies between basic research (which is typically well-funded through grants) and achieving a human proof-of-concept.

Historically, pre-seed and seed capital were the domain of angel investors, although venture capital firms have become increasingly more engaged in recent years.

Series A

Series A is where quantifiable metrics and milestones become the main focus for investors.

Startups with lower regulatory hurdles at this stage are hyper-focused on revenue growth. Sales also takes center stage with investors emphasizing multiple sales channels and new marketing processes. A company's "ideal customer" also comes into focus.

For startups with Class II Medical Devices, Series A funds can be used to apply for 510(k) clearance. Startups developing Class III Medical Devices will require larger amounts of funding to achieve a Pre-Market Approval (PMA) through the FDA, but will use this round to complete the necessary de-risking milestones to achieve regulatory compliance. For drugs, which must go through a lengthy and expensive drug approval process, Series A funds are often used for Investigational New Drug (IND) application submission and sometimes completion of Phase I human clinical trials.

Series B+

During Series B rounds, not only should product/market fit be clearly established, but funding is typically geared toward moving the company from proven to scaled. Subsequent "Series" rounds of financing are where the game elevates into large-scale expansion - whether into international markets or through potential acquisitions. Companies with higher regulatory burdens can use these subsequent rounds of funding to finance the completion of regulatory requirements, which often include completing large-scale clinical trials.

Initial Public Offering (IPO)

At this stage, a company has fully matured with a clear roadmap to success. As a result the founders/investors have opted to take the company to the next level by making shares public to outside investors. IPO funding provides access to new capital that can advance the company beyond the limits of private capital. This is especially crucial for companies that need to raise upward of hundreds of millions of dollars to get through Phase 3 clinical trials or PMA approval for medical devices. Another benefit of an IPO is that it presents an exit opportunity for the earlier stage investors.

Case Study: Invenio Imaging Inc.
Surgical Innovation Startup Hits Funding Milestones

What began as a multi-disciplinary collaboration between a chemist, physicist and neurosurgeon has led to a thriving bioscience business that has navigated the funding process from the initial grant-stage to its current attempt to secure Series B funds for commercialization.

Invenio Imaging Inc. was founded in 2012 based on research from the group of Professor Sunney Xie of the Department of Chemistry and Chemical Biology at Harvard University. Invenio delivered the first fully integrated Stimulated Raman Scattering (SRS) research microscope to the group of Dr. Daniel Orringer at the University of Michigan Department of Neurosurgery thanks to non-dilutive funding, including grants from the National Science Foundation (NSF), Small Business Innovation Research (SBIR) Program, the National Institutes of Health (NIH) Bioengineering Research Partnership Program, and the University of Michigan Translational Research and Commercialization (MTRAC) initiative. The system has been validated at Michigan Medicine on samples from over 800 patients. With additional funding from the NIH SBIR program, an NIBIB bioengineering partnership R01 and an NCI academic industrial partnership R01 they developed the first clinical Stimulated Raman Histology (SRH) imaging system, which is a technology for the non-destructive microscopic analysis of the molecular make-up of tissues and other materials.

In addition to the grant-based infusions, Invenio raised a $1 million Seed round and a $3 million Series A, both of which were led by Mission Bay Capital and included the University of Michigan MINTS as an investor. The next funding milestone for the company will be a $10 million Series B round that will be devoted to commercialization.

Behind the Money

Knowledge is power and the more a healthcare entrepreneur knows about the various avenues for capital, the better prepared they will be when pursuing the appropriate avenue for their start-ups (Table 5.2).

Table 5.2 Healthcare investors

Investor	Description	Examples
Friends & family	The name says it all. Often the first step for passionate investors as they attempt to launch their endeavor.	Personal friends and close relatives
Incubators	Incubators nurture startups in a variety of ways, including providing a space to work in a collaborative environment, seed funding, mentoring, training and other benefits.	Matter, JLABS, Rock Health, StartUp Health
Accelerators	Accelerators are fixed-term, cohort-based programs that include seed investment, connections, mentorship, educational components, and culminate in a public pitch event or demo day to accelerate growth.	Blueprint Health, Dreamit HealthTech, Health Wildcatters, StartX Med, Techstars Healthcare Accelerator, Y Combinator
Crowdfunding	One of the new kids on the block in the investment world, crowdfunding typically involves raising money from a large amount of small investors via the internet. This is becoming more popular as doctors are joining platforms to fund other doctors.	AngelList, AngelMD, FundRx, MedStartr
Angels	Angel investors can be a single person or a group of high net worth individuals who tend to support regional startups through the difficult early stages.	BlueWater Angels, Grand Angels, Life Science Angels, Mid Atlantic Bio Angels, MD Angels, New York Angels, Woodward Angels
Venture capital	Venture Capital firms professionally manage funds raised from limited partners by deploying capital into emerging private companies. VC firms differentiate themselves by their industry focus, check size, and risk-appetite (early-stage vs late-stage).	Arboretum Ventures, Bessemer Venture Partners, BioStar Ventures, Cambia Health, Excel Venture Management, First Round Capital, GV (formerly Google Ventures), Khosla Ventures, New Enterprise Associates, Rock Health
Family offices	Family offices manage the assets of wealthy families and individuals. Whereas these entities once relied on others to invest in startup opportunities on their behalf, in recent years family offices have become more proactive in advancing their own investment aims.	Modi Investment Group, Stetson Family Office, The Paliwoda Group

(continued)

Table 5.2 (continued)

Investor	Description	Examples
Venture philanthropy	Foundations and patient groups are starting to take a more direct approach toward finding treatments for specific diseases by making investments in small biotech companies -- a shift from their traditional approach of funding basic research at universities.	CureDuchenne Ventures, Cystic Fibrosis Foundation, JDRF T1D Fund
Corporate venture funds	Backed by pharmaceutical giants, insurance companies and other corporations, corporate venture firms typically invest in companies with disruptive potential and with an eye toward strategic partnerships.	BlueCross BlueShield Venture Partners, Kaiser Permanente Ventures, Medtronic Ventures, Novartis Venture Fund, Philips Ventures, Sanofi Ventures
Private equity	Private equity firms typically buy a majority stake, up to 100% ownership, of mature companies that are already established.	Aquiline Capital Partners, BlueMountain Capital Management, Clayton, Dubilier & Rice, KKR & Co., Platinum Equity, Summit Partners, Veritas Capital
Hedge funds	Hedge funds are aggressively managed portfolios that use alternative investment strategies in an effort to protect investment portfolios from market uncertainty, while generating high returns in both up and down markets.	Baker Bros. Advisors, Broadfin Capital, DAFNA Capital, EcoR1 Capital, RA Capital
Investment banks	Investment banks assist in raising financial capital, advising companies involved in mergers and acquisitions (M&A), and providing ancillary services such as market making, and trading of derivatives and equity securities.	Bank of America/Merrill Lynch, Cowen Inc., Credit Suisse, Goldman Sachs, JP Morgan, Lazard Capital Markets, Leerink, Oppenheimer, Piper Jaffray, RBC Capital Markets, UBS

Funding Tips for Medpreneurs

1. Nail the "quadruple aim"

   Often used as an investor roadmap, the "quadruple aim" seeks to find health-care innovations that (1) improve the patient experience, (2) improve the care-giver experience, (3) improve health care outcomes, and (4) significantly lower cost.

2. Score "smart" investors

   Smart in this context refers to investors who clearly understand what a company is trying to accomplish and can help partner on strategy and subject matter. Without question, the healthcare arena is complicated and entrepreneurs want investors who understand not only their technology, but also the market in which they hope to thrive.

3. Embrace the headache

    No one wins in the bioscience game without going through the regulatory process. The FDA regulatory landscape is notoriously complicated and lengthy. Have a realistic goal for what you can accomplish when and be clear with investors about your timeline.

4. Stack your bench

    Build a team that will wow investors who often place more weight on a team's ability to execute rather than the technology itself. While physicians can bring the clinical subject matter expertise to a surgical innovation, there are immense opportunities to work with colleagues across multiple disciplines who bring additionally valuable skills to the table.

5. Watch your back

    Intellectual property is vital. Healthcare entrepreneurs must work with a tech transfer office or an IP attorney to have a solid patent strategy. As soon as a company's "secret sauce" is presented publicly it becomes prior art, so individuals must be careful when presenting new data at conferences or publishing in peer-reviewed journals without protecting their findings first.

6. Work the room

    Money isn't going to fall out of the sky. Attend startup-specific networking events to build a solid foundation of investor and industry contacts. Leverage your contacts by following up with them. The old adage is true, "If you want money, ask for advice, and if you want advice, ask for money."

7. Know your worth

    Valuing your company too low and giving away too much equity may leave you with less drive to work hard. Conversely, valuing your company too high may drive away value-added investors and increase the chances of raising a "down round" in the future.

8. Know the deal

    How you raise money can be just as important as *how much* you raise. Make sure you understand the nuances between raising via an equity round, convertible note, and SAFE agreement, for example. There are many terms within each of these documents that can be negotiated to favor the incoming investors over the existing shareholders, and vice versa.

9. Remember the investors' end game

    Never forget that investors are ultimately interested in building a company's value and then driving toward an exit, which can be an IPO or an M&A event. No one is in it to lose.

10. Bring your A-game every day

    Entrepreneurship is not for the faint of heart. Winners in this game know that sitting back and expecting a paycheck without hustle is never going to win you favor with investors or ultimately success in the market. Stay driven, stay hungry and ultimately you will not only land on your feet but hopefully your innovations with make a difference to the people that really matter—the patients.

Conclusion

Fundamentally, attracting the right investors at the right time isn't rocket science or even brain surgery. But creating a successful, sustainable, and ultimately valuable company requires the right mix of due diligence, hard work, and business savvy. The same drive and intellect that surgeons employ every day—whether it's in the operating room or laboratory—is required to score with investors in a highly competitive but ripe market.

The competitive edge will go to those surgeons willing to embrace the business world and apply their laser-like focus to building multi-disciplinary and impressive teams while fully managing the risks and seizing the opportunity.

Chapter 6
Relationships Between Industry and Academic Surgery Departments: Where Is the Pendulum Now?

Bruce Gingles and Bruce L. Gewertz

Introduction

The vast majority of medical devices are conceived and tested by practicing physicians with a simple motive - improving care for their own patients. In so doing, physician inventors may increase their professional stature and address their academic goals such as publishing original research and acquiring federal research funding. Successful inventions can also lead to personal monetary rewards such as royalty income or grants of equity in a business. Importantly, surgical and medical innovation is <u>not</u> a zero-sum game where the advantage derived by one party comes at the expense of another; as the adage goes "a rising tide does indeed lift all boats." Delivering better patient care and outcomes confers a broad halo effect whereby the patient, the inventor, the hospital, the community, the manufacturer, and the insurer all benefit in proportion to the total value of the invention.

B. Gingles
Global Technology Assessment and Health Policy, Cook Medical Holdings,
Bloomington, IN, USA
e-mail: Bruce.Gingles@CookMedical.com

B. L. Gewertz (✉)
Department of Surgery, Interventional Services at Cedars-Sinai Health System,
Los Angeles, CA, USA
e-mail: Bruce.Gewertz@cshs.org

© Springer Nature Switzerland AG 2019
M. S. Cohen, L. Kao (eds.), *Success in Academic Surgery: Innovation and Entrepreneurship*, Success in Academic Surgery,
https://doi.org/10.1007/978-3-030-18613-5_6

Background

A typical path for innovation was followed by Issam I. Raad, MD, from the University of Texas, MD Anderson Cancer Center and Rabih O. Darouiche, MD from the Baylor College of Medicine and the Houston Veterans Administration Hospital [1]. On March 11, 1992, they filed a patent for antibiotic combinations that, when applied to device surfaces, reduced embedded gram-positive bacterial colonies more effectively than systemic antibiotics. The patent covered a combination of rifampin and minocycline or rifampin and novobiocin and had the potential to substantially change the course of central venous catheter-related infections [2–4]. The United States Patent and Trademark Office issued their patent, 5217493, on June 8, 1993, just over a year after filing [5].

Patents are a testimony to ingenuity. But the formal recognition of a sufficiently distinctive invention is not enough for many altruistic physicians. More than anything else, Raad and Darouiche were motivated by their deep commitment to improve patient outcomes by reducing the number and severity of device-related bloodstream infections. In short, they wanted to make an impact through their innovation. Success in this final objective is measured by the degree of utilization of an invention and is defined not by the ingenuity or characteristics of the invention, but by the market.

Raad and Darouiche quickly realized that to make their invention into a meaningful clinical tool, they needed a commercial partner to develop an industrial process to reliably adhere the antibiotics to catheters and then, once regulatory approval was achieved, to manufacture and market the product. The partner they selected was Cook Critical Care, a division of Cook Medical, based in Bloomington, Indiana. In exchange for a license to the patent, jointly owned by Baylor and the University of Texas, Cook agreed to pay the universities a royalty, that in turn, was shared with the inventors and their laboratories per institutional rules.

This is hardly a new or unique narrative. Perhaps no story better reveals the remarkable impact such academic-industrial partnerships can have than the discovery and commercialization of insulin by University of Western Ontario surgeon Frederick Banting and University of Toronto physicians Charles Best and J.J.R. Macleod [6].

Researching treatment for diabetes in 1920, Banting and Best discovered that administering insulin to pancreatectomized dogs was curative for the surgically-induced diabetes in these animals. They used their laboratory to extract and purify insulin from mountains of pancreas they obtained from pigs. Ten thousand pounds of raw pancreas were required to produce a single pound of purified insulin. After dramatic and early success, they gradually found they were not able to maintain consistency in the extraction process and their diabetic dogs began to die.

Desperate for access to high quality insulin, they persuaded the University to license their patent to Eli Lilly & Company; where earlier entreaties from Lilly and other drug companies had been rejected. Lilly's newly appointed research director, Dr. George Henry Alexander Clowes, quickly bridged the gap between the University of Toronto's research laboratories and Lilly's industrial facilities. Banting presented his first paper on the success of their operations and insulin injections in 1921. By 1923, Lilly was selling insulin to hospitals and clinics across North America [7]. Almost immediately, the implications of a diagnosis of diabetes were dramatically changed from suffering and death to prolonged survival and relative health.

The inventors were feted and revered for life. Banting and Macleod won the Noble prize in 1923; Banting split the monetary prize with Best. The investigators were granted a lifetime annuity to continue their research. In 1934, Frederick Banting was knighted by King George V.

Given this extraordinary history and the numerous examples of other successful industrial-academic partnerships over the last 100 years, it is puzzling that there has been such venomous criticism of industry's financial support of inventors and clinical researchers in both popular media and peer-reviewed medical journals. A highly negative JAMA report in 1986 [8] steeled the resolve of medical schools [9], regulators [10], medical societies [11], and many medical journals [12] toward more regulated relationships between industry and physicians. The resulting climate of general disapproval of such collaborative activities has tarnished even routine commercial practices like product marketing, which is essential to speed adoption and recover the investments made in developing new therapies. This negative posture is remarkable when considering that during this period, medicine saw the launch of innumerable pioneering advances such as angioplasty, stenting, diagnostic ultrasound, and minimally invasive surgery; all of which have greatly impacted both life expectancy and quality of life [7, 13].

Our Argument for Strong Partnerships Between Academic and Industrial Entities

While we would agree that there are challenges and potential pitfalls in every relationship, it is our contention that the benefits of industrial-academic partnerships far exceed the problems. A number of surveys indicate that this favorable opinion appears to be held by most academic physicians.

In 2009, questionnaires were mailed to 515 randomly selected physicians in the American College of Obstetricians and Gynecologists' Collaborative Ambulatory Research Network [14]. Recipients were queried about their reliance on pharmaceutical sales representatives for product information and samples; nearly half of the physicians (251) responded. Despite the fact that 62% of respondents had read guidelines discouraging interaction between physicians and industry, 71% still used sales representatives for help with prescribing.

Another survey in 2010 captured input from 590 physicians and medical students [15]. Sixty-five percent agreed with the statement: "pharmaceutical company materials are useful for learning about new drugs." When asked whether, "device company materials are useful for learning about new devices," 78% agreed while 71%

endorsed the statement that "pharmaceutical and device company funds are useful for funding medical school programs." Importantly, only the minority of resident-student respondents (33%) and faculty (23%) agreed that "my institution should prohibit resident-student or attending interactions with pharmaceutical and device company representatives."

A meta-analysis of available opinion surveys, published in 2011, suggested that students generally did <u>not</u> support excluding sales representatives or industry presentations from the learning environment [16]. Furthermore, when looking forward to the next step of their career, 86% of American medical students reported that they would wish to interact with pharmaceutical sales representatives during their residencies. Despite these results, the authors were undeterred from what appeared to be a predetermined conclusion, echoing the general attitude opposing academic-industrial interactions. They closed with a recommendation best characterized as a non-sequitur: "Interventions that decrease students' contact with industry and eliminate gifts may have a positive effect on building the "healthy skepticism" that evidence-based medical practice requires."

This prevailing attitude has been rebutted, albeit modestly, over the last 25 years. A range of counter-balancing voices have pointed out the considerable benefits of industrial-academic partnerships including the development, testing and promulgation of path-breaking medicines (e.g. statins) and innovative treatments for valvular and vascular disease (e.g. cardiovascular prostheses) [17–19].

Endovascular grafting for aortic aneurysms is a prime example familiar to the authors. More than 90% of all infrarenal aneurysms are now treated with endovascular techniques rather than open surgical repair [20]. This remarkable conversion occurred over a brief 10-year period, overcoming all geographic and financial barriers. Thanks to educational programs, which often partnered academic medical centers with graft manufacturers, virtually all practicing vascular surgeons and interventional cardiologists who desired the skill set were able to learn endografting.

While the rapid expansion of this treatment can be directly attributed to the unquestioned reduction in perioperative morbidity and mortality, adoption of endografts for nearly all aneurysms also reflects the relentless development of safe, reliable devices that are adaptable to wide variations in anatomy. Is there any conceivable path by which this truly transformative technology would have developed so quickly without the strong support of a medical device industry stimulated by the upside of increasing their market share and gaining a fair return on investment?

All that said, we are aware of both real and potential conflicts of interest. Early trials of new devices often involve physicians who are enthusiastic about the procedure, even if the actual inventors of the device may be excluded from supervisory roles in the clinical tests. Without question, the attention gained from introducing new and effective treatments increases both the local stature of the "pioneering" physician and provides material for noteworthy publications that enhance their national recognition. This advantage is counterbalanced by the potential diminution in reputation if a physician too often introduces treatments that are eventually shown to be ill-advised or even harmful. As the ancient maxim warns "you don't get unlimited bites of the apple."

Another mandate that should be acknowledged is the absolute requirement for full disclosure of any proprietary interests (including stock ownership or advisory fees) when authoring a report in peer-reviewed journals. This directive applies to all academic exercises, including invited journal reviews of clinical reports from others who use the specific device that the reviewer has an interest in. This caveat is equally important when clinical opinion leaders are reviewing results from competing manufacturers who are offering an alternative device. At times, the safest path is recusal to avoid any appearance of bias.

If you were to accept our hypothesis that some substantial fraction of medical progress depends on commercialization of innovations from practicing physicians, the logical next step would be assessing the barriers to this process and how those could be mitigated without violating ethical norms. Below, we will outline three of the most important threats to innovation, one in each stage of development.

The most critical *early* challenge relates to the surgeon's role in conceiving and clinically validating their own invention Historically, once physicians imagined a potentially better solution to a significant clinical problem, they would then recruit a manufacturer to prototype, test, develop, and produce the invention. Such new devices cannot be used in patients in the USA until they are cleared or approved by the Federal Food and Drug Administration (FDA) or have been registered in a clinical trial under an Investigational Device Exemption (IDE). By the time new devices reach patients, they have already been determined by FDA to be safe and effective or they have been found to present minimal risk through the Pre-Market Notification system, also known as class II devices, the most common being a 510(k) regulatory pathway. For the overwhelming majority of 510(k)-cleared devices, the first clinical cases represent product evaluation, not research.

The innovator's role in product evaluation and refinement is vital. In the initial stages, the majority of product design and clinical performance input rightfully comes from this single individual. Clinical feedback provided to the manufacturer by the inventor prior to broad commercialization is a next vital step to ensure that every nuance of the product meets the inventor's strict design requirements. This evaluation phase permits refinement of even the smallest attributes unsatisfactory to the inventor. The influence on product design and performance is so great that it is common in the device industry, unlike pharmaceuticals, for the product to be named after the inventor. Fabled inventors such as Fogarty, Foley, Swan-Ganz, Gruentzig, Arndt, Ciaglia, Gianturco, Cope and Amplatz are only a few examples [21–25].

In days long past, it was customary for inventors to not only conduct the initial clinical evaluations but also to report their early experience in peer-reviewed journals. Today, as a means of mitigating conflicts of interest, academic surgeons are often prohibited by department chairs or deans from evaluating their own inventions. While this removes any bias, it robs manufacturers of the vital feedback that only someone intimately familiar with the device (i.e. the inventor) can provide.

   B. Gingles and B. L. Gewertz

In substitution, "disinterested" medically-qualified third parties may be assigned to perform preliminary cases and to share their comments. Problems often occur if minor specifications such as length, trigger tension, ergonomics or even color need adjusting. If these limitations are initially displeasing to the evaluator, the prototype is often discarded with only cursory reports to the engineer. In sum without the passion of the inventor, the truly "neutral" surrogate is all too often content to return to the familiar standard rather than insisting on a design change. The most common and damning sentiment is "it's not really any better than our current approach." The engineer is substantially disadvantaged from this chain of events; there is simply no "true source" for the ideal except the inventor.

An ethical, transparent, and practical remedy lies in the direct participation of the inventor in the evaluation of their product, under the watchful eye of an independently appointed, medically qualified "chaperone" who is not authoritatively subordinated to the inventor. The chaperone's two critical roles are to (1) rigorously review candidates for the procedure to ensure all are appropriately selected and properly indicated and (2) be present during the performance of all procedures to assure fidelity of procedure/incident reporting and to insist that adherence to proper surgical standards are maintained. If any irregularities are observed, these are reported directly to the service chief or chair for remediation. At least one large academic medical center has successfully employed this policy [26].

Based on our combined experience, we would generally discount concern about conflicted inventors racing their technologies to market and into the untrained hands of physicians. After their initial experiences with commercialization, the mature inventor is deeply aware of the years and money spent bringing their technology through innumerable pre-market milestones. They are also clear about the disastrous consequences of even a single serious complication during early phases of commercialization; one or two bad outcomes are enough to ruin years of hard work.

A second and insidious challenge to surgical innovation arises in the *later* stages, when products become commercially available The primary and overarching motive for surgeon inventors is to elevate the care of their patients. It is the rational expectation of clinical inventors that once products are sold in the market, their hospital will make these available through supply chain functions so that their patients and the hospital can benefit from the rewards that flow from better outcomes. Indeed, a common litmus test by device manufacturers when considering proposals from clinical inventors is to ask, "If we invest in your technology, will you use it on your own patients once the device becomes commercially available?"

It is now common for surgeons to see their product enter the market only to be told by their own hospital that the product will not be purchased and made available either to the inventor or other physicians at their hospital. This is particularly discouraging after years of hard work and sacrifice. The reasons for denial are many, including binding supply contracts with competitors, financial penalties to the institution for deviating from Group Purchasing Organization (GPO) compliance agreements, the nuisance of inventory conversion requiring inter-departmental staff training and, of course, the perception of conflicts of interest.

To mitigate the perception of inappropriate commercial incentives, manufacturers have increasingly withheld royalties from whole institutions at which physician-inventors treat patients. While practical in theory, accurate royalty tracking is often unreliable due to complex supply chain processes, including ubiquitous intermediary product handlers. Further, when inventors are prevented from using their own technologies, the device easily moves to neighboring hospitals unburdened by such concerns. In an ironic twist, the inventor and/or their institution is actually placed in competition against the invention, and this is not a rare event today.

This situation also presents a special challenge to manufacturers. Building a brand around an inventor's device relies heavily on confidence created in the market that the inventor is customer "number one." This is especially true if the product carries the inventor's name. Inquisitive, prospective customers frequently want to know about the inventor's experience with their device before committing to adoption. Any failure of the inventor to accumulate cases and share their results is an impediment to market adoption for that medical innovation and is not easily explained nor overcome.

To our mind the refusal by a hospital or academic medical center to acquire their faculty's products is a substantial challenge to innovation Hospitals have reasonable leverage when their faculty develop better methods of care. Cost is almost never the issue since manufacturers have every incentive to ensure that inventors are active users. Companies generally reflect that imperative within supply chain agreements and purchasing contracts. One increasingly popular tool for managing the risk of adopting unproven medical technologies is the Performance-Based Risk Sharing Agreement (PBRSA). PBRSAs synchronize price and product performance; such that as greater performance is realized, price is increased, thereby modulating risk between the buyer and seller. For innovators, it is prudent to know their hospital's policies toward homegrown technology as early as possible. If the institution is ideologically resistant, and the invention is key to their personal and professional satisfaction, there is often no choice but to transfer to another, more accommodating environment.

The final challenge to successful academic – industrial partnerships is cultural in nature and reflects poorly considered institutional policies that inhibit transparent and proper interactions Certain medical societies and universities work with a mental model in which industry and medicine are occupants of distinct but parallel moral universes, never to be intertwined. As an example of this thinking, in 2005, the Journal of the American Medical Association (JAMA) issued a directive requiring that industry-sponsored studies be submitted to separate and independent statistical analysis by a non-involved biostatistician [27]. No such secondary analysis was required of papers funded by other sources. In 2013, the policy was reversed, with JAMA claiming, "our experience has been that the conduct of additional analyses by independent academic biostatisticians generally did not result in meaningful changes in study results." JAMA further stated, "Advances over the past decade in standards of clinical trial reporting, enhanced understanding of the threats to validity of clinical research, increasing data transparency, and our experience support the change in policy." [28]

In 2010, the American Heart Association (AHA) announced a policy prohibiting any industry employee from poster or oral presentations at AHA meetings. Backlash from the scientific and clinical communities was rapid and fierce, resulting in prompt and embarrassing retraction [29]. Had this policy been allowed to move forward, acknowledged experts, including Nobel laureates like Philip Sharp (Biogen), Richard Roberts (New England Biolabs) and Ferid Murad (Abbott), would be barred from addressing their peers at AHA conferences [30].

Conclusion

Innovation in academic medical centers by employed faculty is a national asset and a crucial pathway for improving patient care. Meaningful interactions with industry are essential to develop and refine new technologies, produce them in scale, and shepherd them through the rigorous regulatory processes. Finally, without the marketing and sales support of device and pharmaceutical companies, even meritorious inventions and molecules would not make the kind of positive impact on outcomes that patients deserve.

While there will always be potential conflicts of both effort and interest, we continue to believe these can best be addressed through thoughtful accommodations in a spirit of compromise rather than overarching proclamations suggesting mal-intent. The process of medical innovation is simply too important to impede.

Conflicts of Interest The ideas and opinions expressed herein are those of the authors and may not reflect, in whole or in part, the position of Cook Medical Holdings, LLC.

References

1. Raad I, Darouiche R, Dupuis J, et al. Central venous catheters coated with minocycline and rifampin for the prevention of catheter-related colonization and bloodstream infections. Ann Intern Med. 1997;127:267–74.
2. Hanna HA, Radd II, Hackett B, et al. Antibiotic-impregnated catheters associated with significant decrease in nosocomial and multidrug-resistant bacteremias in critically ill patients. Chest. 2003;124:1030–8.
3. Bonne S, Mazuski JE, Sona C, et al. Effectiveness of minocycline and rifampin vs chlorhexidine and silver sulfadiazine-impregnated central venous catheters in preventing central line-associated bloodstream infection in a high-volume academic intensive care unit: a before and after trial. J Am Coll Surg. 2015;221:739–47.
4. Darouiche RO, Raad II, Heard SO, et al. A comparison of two antimicrobial-impregnated central venous catheters. N Engl J Med. 1999;340:1–8.
5. USPTO patent number 5217493.

6. Cooper T, Ainsberg A. Breakthrough: Elizabeth Hughes, the discovery of insulin and the making of a medical miracle: St. Marten's Press; 2010.
7. https://www.seniorliving.org/history/1900-2000-changes-life-expectancy-united-states/. Accessed 31 Oct 18.
8. Brennan TA, Rothman D, Blank L, et al. Health industry practices that create conflicts of interest. JAMA. 2006;295(4):429–33.
9. Korn D, Carlat D. Conflicts of interest in medical education. JAMA. 2004;310:2397–8.
10. ACCME Standards for commercial support. https://www.accme.org/publications/accme-standards-for-commercial-support. Accessed 31 Oct 18.
11. https://cmss.org/wp-content/uploads/2016/02/CMSS-Code-for-Interactions-with-Companies-Approved-Revised-Version-4.13.15-with-Annotations.pdff. Accessed 31 Oct 18.
12. https://jamanetwork.com/journals/jama/fullarticle/1216459. Accessed 31 Oct 18.
13. Lichtenberg F. The impact of biomedical innovation on longevity and health. Nordic J Healt Econ. 2017;5:45–57.
14. Anderson B, Lowenstein G, Schulkin J, et al. Factors associated with physicians' reliance on pharmaceutical sales representatives. Acad Med. 2009;84:994–1002.
15. Korenstein D, Salomeh K, Ross J. Physicians attitudes toward industry. Arch Surg. 2010;145(6):570–7.
16. Austad KE, Avorn J, Kesselheim AS. Medical students' exposure to and attitudes about the pharmaceutical industry: a systematic review. PLoS Med. https://journals.plos.org/plosmedicine/article?id=10.1371/journal.pmed.1001037. Accessed 31 Oct 18. 2011;8:e1001037.
17. Rothman KJ. Conflict of interest: the new McCarthyism in science. JAMA. 1993;269:2782–4.
18. Stossel TP. Pharmaphobia: Rowman & Littlefield; 2015.
19. Rosenbaum L. Reconnecting the dots-reinterpreting industry-physician relations. NEJM. 2015;372:1860–4.
20. Ng T, Mirocha J, Magner D, Gewertz BL. Regional variations in the utilization of endovascular aneurysm repair reflect population risk factors and disease prevalence. J Vasc Surg. 2010;51:801–9.
21. Thal AP, Quick KL. A guided chest tube for safe thoracostomy. Surg Gynecol Obstet. 1988;167:517.
22. Ciaglia P, Firsching R, Syniec C. Elective percutaneous dilatational tracheostomy. A new simple bedside procedure; preliminary report. Chest. 1985;87:715–9.
23. Fuhrman BP, Landrum BG, Ferrara TB, et al. Pleural drainage using modified pigtail catheters. Crit Care Med. 1986;14:575–6.
24. Lock JE, Bass JL, Kulil TJ, et al. Chronic percutaneous drainage with modified pigtail catheters in children. Am J Cardiol. 1984;53:1179–82.
25. Sargent EN, Turner F. Emergency treatment of pneumothorax. Am J Roentgenol Rad Therapy Nuclear Med. 1970;109:531–5.
26. Ross McKinney, MD, personal communication. Accessed 31 Oct 18.
27. Fontarosa PB, Flanigan A, DeAngelis CD. Reporting conflicts of interest, financial aspects of research, and role of sponsors in funded studies. JAMA. 2005;294:110–1.
28. Bauchner H. Editorial policies for clinical trials and the continued changes in medical journalism. JAMA. 2013;310(2):149–50.
29. https://www.policymed.com/2010/06/aha-ban-on-industry-posters-and-presenters-conflict-of-interest-run-amuck.html. Accessed 31 Oct 18.
30. http://www.nobel.se/medicine/laureates/1998/murad-autobio.html, https://www.nobelprize.org/prizes/medicine/1998/murad/auto-biography. Accessed 31 Oct 18.

Chapter 7
The Biodesign Model: Training Physician Innovators and Entrepreneurs

Dimitri A. Augustin, Lyn Denend, James Wall, Thomas Krummel, and Dan E. Azagury

Biodesign Model

Stanford Biodesign was founded in 2000 by Dr. Paul Yock, an interventional cardiologist and inventor. His goal was to create an ecosystem of training and support for Stanford University students, fellows, and faculty with the talent and ambition to become leaders in health technology innovation. In collaboration with entrepreneur Josh Makower, Yock launched the Biodesign Innovation Fellowship in 2001—a first-of-its-kind, one-year, full-time training program for aspiring innovators with backgrounds in medicine, engineering, and business. In 2005, Dr. Tom Krummel, a pediatric surgeon, joined the team to introduce Biodesign to surgeons during their research years. Over time, the Biodesign approach expanded beyond Stanford

D. A. Augustin
Division of Nephrology, Department of Medicine, Stanford University, Stanford, CA, USA

Stanford Byers Center for Biodesign, Stanford University, Stanford, CA, USA
e-mail: daa1@stanford.edu

L. Denend
Stanford Byers Center for Biodesign, Stanford University, Stanford, CA, USA
e-mail: denend@stanford.edu

J. Wall · T. Krummel
Stanford Byers Center for Biodesign, Stanford University, Stanford, CA, USA

Division of Pediatric Surgery, Department of Surgery, Stanford University, Stanford, CA, USA
e-mail: jkwall@stanford.edu; tkrummel@stanford.edu

D. E. Azagury (✉)
Stanford Byers Center for Biodesign, Stanford University, Stanford, CA, USA

Department of Surgery, Stanford University, Stanford, CA, USA
e-mail: dazagury@stanford.edu

© Springer Nature Switzerland AG 2019
M. S. Cohen, L. Kao (eds.), *Success in Academic Surgery: Innovation and Entrepreneurship*, Success in Academic Surgery,
https://doi.org/10.1007/978-3-030-18613-5_7

University and is now widely taught within universities, institutions, and corporations across the United States and around the world.

At the heart of the Stanford Biodesign approach is the "biodesign innovation process" –a comprehensive, repeatable process for need-driven health technology innovation. The process is based on the design thinking methodology, but also incorporates specific activities that are essential for bringing a new invention forward in the complex healthcare environment. Following the approach, innovators identify compelling unmet clinical needs, invent novel solutions to address them, and prepare to implement those new medical devices, diagnostics, and other technologies into patient care, with the hope of improving outcomes and/or reducing costs to the healthcare system. The process has been adopted by innovators at the undergraduate, graduate, post-graduate, and executive levels. However, this chapter will focus specifically on how physician innovators and entrepreneurs can engage in this process and apply it to their careers.

Components of the Biodesign Innovation Process

The Biodesign innovation process includes three phases: identify, invent, and implement. Each phase has two stages that are supported by a total of 29 core activities (Fig. 7.1).

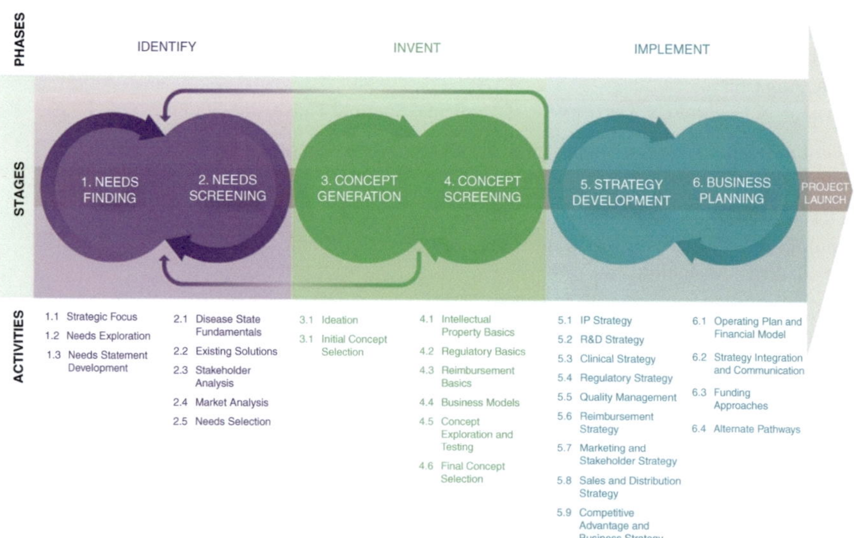

Fig. 7.1 The Biodesign Process. Source: Stanford Biodesign (reprinted with permission)

Identify

The identify phase is the first and most critical part of the biodesign innovation process. Rather than taking a technology-driven approach to invention, where the innovator makes an interesting technological discovery and then seeks to find a problem it can be used to solve, the Stanford Biodesign method is need-driven (needs are roughly defined as opportunities for innovation). Innovators begin by deeply understanding and evaluating what unmet clinical needs exist in their area of focus. Only once they have become "expert" in the most compelling needs do they take what they have learned and apply it to coming up with a unique solution. In an environment where new health technologies can take 5–10 years and hundreds of millions of dollars to bring into patient care, this targeted approach can be more efficient than the discovery model. The identify phase includes stage 1: needs finding and stage 2: needs screening.

Needs Finding

Needs finding begins with choosing a strategic focus for their innovation effort. This requires innovators to first explore their own values, assets, strengths, and weaknesses to create objective "acceptance criteria" for deciding in which subject areas to seek innovation projects. Innovators look at a variety of opportunity areas: their medical specialty, related interest areas, research and data that captures their attention, and their personal passion. Additionally, external factors beyond the innovator's direct control may sway focus decisions. For example, an unpredictable reimbursement landscape or risk-averse climate in a particular area of medicine may steer one away from that space. Innovators evaluate all of these inputs to define individual or team acceptance criteria (e.g., project should result in a new technology that is life-saving rather than life-enhancing; project should be realizable in 7 years or less). In turn, they use these criteria to assess innovation opportunities to determine which ones offer a strong fit. Importantly, acceptance criteria are unique to every innovator or team (there is no right or wrong answer!). Additionally, some opportunities will not align with an innovator's acceptance criteria at a particular point in time, but that fit may evolve over time as the innovator's situation, team, environment, and expertise change.

Once a strategic focus area has been chosen, innovators begin needs finding by immersing themselves directly in the daily activities of the focus area being studied. During this immersion, innovators perform direct observations across the relevant cycle of care, making note of unmet clinical needs. They then actively refine their observations through background research and focused interviews with those involved in the cycle of care. This information helps the innovators corroborate or invalidate assumptions made during the direct observations.

For each validated observation, the innovators next generate **need statements**, which are fundamental to the biodesign innovation process. Need statements are one sentence "mission statements" that capture the essence of the need. Each one is made up of three essential components: the clinical problem, the population it affects, and the targeted change in outcome. For example, "a way to detect rhythm disturbances [problem] in non-hospitalized patients with suspected arrhythmias [population] to improve the patient experience and reduce the cost of diagnosis [outcome]." The original need statement will undergo multiple iterations as more information about the need is uncovered. Through an exercise called need scoping, innovators experiment with different versions of the need statement – making the problem, population, and/or outcome broader or more focused – until they find the one that is best supported by their research and validation interviews. In parallel, they choose each word in the need statement carefully since minor variations in wording can send the innovators in significantly different directions for the rest of the design process.

One common pitfall in creating a need statement is embedding a solution into it. This mistake artificially constrains the innovation project by linking it to an existing technology paradigm. For example, a need for "a stent that prevents vessel wall material from embolizing…" is much more limited than one that defines the problem as "a way to prevent the consequences of emboli secondary to an interventional procedure…" With the first example, the team will be restricted to thinking about how to engineer a better stent. With the second, they can explore a much greater range of possible solutions.

Needs Screening

The needs screening stage is the second part of the identify phase. During needs finding, innovators seek to identify and understand many needs. During needs screening, their objective is to evaluate those needs to identify the one(s) that represent the most promising innovation opportunities to take forward into the invent phase. This is accomplished by making the needs "compete" against one another on a series of objective factors and then choosing the ones that perform the best. The specific screening factors are defined by each innovator or team. They take into account the acceptance criteria defined earlier, but also include factors such as the number of patients affected, the severity of the unaddressed problem, the extent to which key stakeholders believe a new solution is needed, and the size of the potential market.

In order to evaluate each need against the defined screening factors, innovators conduct significantly more need research in four key areas: disease state, existing solutions, stakeholders, and market analysis. Disease state analysis involves an in-depth review of the disease epidemiology, anatomy and physiology, pathophysiology, clinical presentation, clinical outcomes, and economic impact. A full review of existing solutions for a given need helps an innovator not only understand what treatments, diagnostics, or other interventions are currently available, but where gaps may exist in the current care system. It is also important to consider what new solutions are in development or testing that may alter the competitive landscape.

Stakeholder analysis is particularly important since the adoption of medical innovations is dependent on multiple individuals and groups. There are two common approaches for identifying all of the stakeholders involved in a specific need area. The first is cycle of care analysis, which breaks down the cycle of care from diagnosis through treatment and follow up, and then identifies all of the individuals involved and the different roles they play. The second approach is to look at the flow of money in the need area to understand who participates and how they are financially rewarded. Oftentimes, different stakeholders have different interests that influence their decision to adopt a new technology. Patients, for example, might be most concerned about sustaining or improving their quality of life. Physicians are often most interested in new technologies with the potential to improve clinical outcomes, but they also might consider how their workflow is affected, the complications their patients endure, or the frustrations they experience with the current standard of care. Facilities are motivated by how a new solution might affect the economics of delivering care to the patients they serve, but they also think about other considerations such as how new technologies might enhance their reputation. Payers must consider the health outcomes of the people they insure, as well as their own bottom line. The key is to understand the extent to which each major stakeholder group is likely to embrace or resist a new solution to the need. To organize stakeholder data, innovators can assess the net impact of a new solution as being positive or negative for each group. Innovators should also make note of which stakeholder is the decision maker and which are the influencers.

Common examples of positive and negative impacts to stakeholders with new devices.

Stakeholders	Positive impacts	Negative impacts
Payers	Long-term cost savings for covering a defined population; reduced near-term reimbursement payments	Increased upfront costs
Physicians	Improved patient outcomes; improved workflow; increased revenue for adopters	New training to use device; change in workflow; negative effect on practice if device shifts care to alternate provider
Facilities	Increased revenue; reduced costs; reduced complications/ errors; market advantage/ reputation	Capital expenses; lack of current reimbursement pathway
Patients	Improved quality of life; improved overall health and procedural outcomes; reduction in mortality	Increased out of pocket costs; increased personal risk; lack of access to new technology

Market analysis is performed to estimate what value can be captured in a given need area. The three key steps are market landscaping, market segmentation, and choosing a target market. The market landscaping allows the innovators to evaluate the presence and importance of the market opportunity and estimate the overall current and future size of the addressable market for each need. For market segmentation, the market is divided into multiple groups, further addressing the size and growth, competition, and stakeholder influence in each of those submarkets. The last step, target market, identifies which segment stands to gain the most value from a new solution so that this group may be targeted first if/when a new product is brought into patient care.

Once all of the required research has been gathered, innovators can use it to rate each need against the defined screening factors, calculate a score for each one, and then create a ranking of all the needs under consideration. The needs at the bottom of the list are set aside, while additional research and validation is performed for those at the top. This cycle is typically repeated multiple times until the innovators decide on just a few top needs to take forward into the invent phase of the process.

Importantly, for each of the chosen needs, the innovators use their accumulated research to define "need criteria." Need criteria are those requirements that *any* new solution must be able to satisfy in order to have a chance of being adopted and displacing the current standard of care. Typically, the innovators create 3–4 "must have" and 3–4 "nice to have" criteria that represent the factors that are most important to the stakeholders affected by the need. Sample need criteria might include the target cost for a new technology, its required accuracy rate, the time it takes to use, or other such requirements. In this way, the need criteria provide guidance to the innovators as they prepare to begin ideating and inventing solutions.

Case Study: Identify Phase
Insite Medical

Dr. James Wall, a pediatric surgeon at Stanford University, first thought he wanted to solve problems in medicine during his undergraduate days as a bioengineering student. By the second year of medical school, he was exploring ways to pursue both medicine and engineering. He participated in an engineering in medicine program during medical school but became frustrated by the inability to take the next step and implement a new technology into clinical practice. During his training, he made his way to the West Coast and became a Stanford Biodesign Innovation Fellow in 2006, with the hope of becoming a physician innovator and advancing new medical technologies into patient care.

At the beginning of the fellowship, Dr. Wall and his team members made a series of observations in the operating room of the pediatric hospital. In one case, the patient, pending a procedure for a chest deformity, required epidural anesthesia. They watched as the anesthesiologist struggled to access the epidural space. Through additional background research, they found that epidural complications were rare, but the outcomes from those complications were significant. Furthermore, epidurals routinely caused procedure delays given the complex and variable nature of gaining access in different patients. Dr. Wall and his team summarized their observed problem around getting timely, repeatable epidural access. They evaluated multiple populations including, from largest to smallest, obstetric patients, elective surgery patients, and chronic pain patients. For the outcome, they focused on reducing complications.

After additional research, their resulting need statement was: "A way to more accurately and safely deliver epidural anesthesia in patients requiring pain management to reduce complications." They screened hundreds of needs but this was ultimately the one they decided to take forward into the invent phase of the biodesign innovation process.

Invent

The invent phase is the second part of the biodesign innovation process. This is when inventors start thinking about concepts that might effectively address the given need and need criteria. Invent includes two stages, concept generation and concept selection.

Concept Generation

Concept generation involves using various ideation techniques to come up with new solutions that can potentially address a need. Although ideation can occur in a variety of ways, brainstorming is the classic approach (as outlined in *The Art of Innovation* [1], by Tom Kelly of IDEO) that is most frequently used. This technique instructs innovators to defer judgment, encourage wild ideas, maintain one conversation at the time, build on the ideas of others, and produce a large quantity of ideas. It is expected that brainstorming sessions remain focused and visual. A facilitator may be used to moderate the sessions. Oftentimes, "how might we" questions are generated based on the need statement and need criteria (e.g., How might we detect rhythm disturbances using methods internal to the patient? How might we detect rhythm disturbances using methods external to the patient? etc.). These "how might we" questions become prompts for initiating each brainstorming session. Other approaches include constructive conflict or modified brainstorming situations when most attention is dedicated to discovering the ideas of a key opinion leader.

Ideation is an iterative exercise that should be completed multiple times using different prompts. After each brainstorming session, concepts are organized and grouped into a concept map so that the innovators can see areas where they have robust ideas and other areas that may require additional ideation. Examples of how concept grouping can be done include anatomic location, engineering type, or appeal to influencers.

Once the innovators have generated dozens (or ideally hundreds) of ideas, they start to think about which concepts seem to be the most promising. This is initially done by evaluating each idea against the need criteria. Concepts that seem to have a high likelihood of meeting all of the "must have" need criteria should be advanced. Those that do not should be set aside or taken into additional brainstorming sessions to see how they can be improved. If too many concepts appear that they can satisfy the need criteria, the criteria may be too broad and should be reworked based on additional research.

Concept Screening

Once a promising set of concepts that align with the need criteria have been identified, the innovators move into more rigorous concept screening. This is similar to needs screening in that the concepts "compete" against one another on a series of important factors: intellectual property, regulatory pathway, reimbursement, business model, and technical feasibility.

Intellectual property searches can effectively be based on the problem, structure of the invention, and function of the invention. The key is to determine which solutions are patentable and will have freedom to operate when they reach the market.

With regard to regulation, each concept is evaluated based on its classification and regulatory pathway for the geographic location where it will initially be used. In the US, these requirements are set forth by the Food and Drug Administration, which categorizes devices into class I, II, or III based on their risk level and then evaluates them through three primary pathways: exempt, 510(k), or Premarket Approval (PMA). In Europe, device regulation, known as CE marking, is governed under three European Commission directives. This structure is also risk based and includes class I, IIa, IIb, and III devices.

When assessing reimbursement, it is important to understand the current payment system(s) used in the need area, including procedure and diagnosis coding and coverage determinations for technologies that are paid for through public and private reimbursement. If existing reimbursement codes can be used for a new solution, this can potentially save the innovators significant time and money in establishing payment for their new technology. The pathway to bringing a new innovation to market becomes much more complex if there is not already an established code that can be used; payment is insufficient to cover the new technology; the time and effort of a new code is not worth pursuing; or similar devices are not currently reimbursed. Technologies not reimbursed may be marketed directly to consumers – a growing trend. They might also be paid for directly by providers or institutions as part of their "overhead" costs. All of these factors vary from country to country and should be evaluated specifically for the initial target market.

The next activity during concept screening is to determine what business model would apply to each solution. The business model defines the interface between the customer and the technology and outlines important factors such as the revenue stream, price, and margin structure for the product. Business model types include disposable products, reusable products, implantable products, capital equipment products, services, fee per use, subscriptions, over-the-counter products, prescription products, and physician-sell products. The innovators evaluate the characteristics of their concept to determine the best business model fit. The biodesign innovation process encourages innovators to validate their top business model ideas with potential purchasers before a final one is chosen.

Technical feasibility is determined through concept exploration and testing. During this step, innovators assess the elements of greatest technical risk for each concept by building prototypes and testing them. Innovators should start by addressing the biggest risks that would otherwise prevent implementation of the concept. Innovators can use a ranking system to know which components pose the biggest risk and then evaluate why. Sometimes, this involves consultation with experts in a particular technical area that is essential to the concept. Typically, the biggest risk is formulated into a question that can be answered with a prototype. Prototypes can be works-like models, feels-like models, is-like models, looks-like models, and look-like/is-like models. Each type of model can be used to test and answer different questions that are critical to the overall success of the technology. At this early stage in the development and testing process, it is not necessary to fulfill all need criteria in a single prototype.

Innovators select a final concept once all aspects of concept screening have been considered. There are different methods for accomplishing this, but one common approach is to assign a rating for how risky each concept is relative to its intellectual property, regulatory, reimbursement, business model, and technical feasibility – for example, green for low risk, yellow for moderate risk, and red for high risk. Concepts with mostly red and yellow ratings can be set aside in favor of those with more green and yellow ratings. Importantly, innovators should also reconfirm that the top concept(s) still address the "must have" and "nice to have" need criteria.

Case Study: Invent Phase
InSite Medical

Dr. Wall and his team excitedly headed into brainstorming with their defined need statement: "A way to more accurately and safely deliver epidural anesthesia in patients requiring pain management to reduce complications." One key insight that aided them during ideation involved the natural anatomy of the spine and surrounding structures. The ligamentum flavum, a thick ligament that needs to be crossed before entering into the epidural space, has mechanical properties that would allow a hollow, screw-like mechanism to engage and slowly penetrate by twisting (like a screw) until the epidural space was reached. The controlled engagement of the ligament would avoid anesthesiologists from penetrating too far and prevent complications such as epidural vein bleeds or dural tears.

Through a series of iterative brainstorming sessions, they came up with multiple solutions that, when screened against the need criteria, showed promise. The team then evaluated the concepts on intellectual property, regulatory, reimbursement, business model, and technical feasibility. Ultimately, the team chose to move forward with the screw-like device with the lowest risk profile from their concept screening exercise, with the hope that it would make epidural access for regional anesthesia safer and more effective, with fewer complications. Dr. Wall explained the concept this way: "With the existing approach, the physician would advance a sharp needle to the ligamentum flavum, which was quite dense. They knew they had reached the right spot when the needle would pop through the other side of the ligament. But they'd have to stop quickly and retract the needle slightly to prevent any unintended injury to the patient. Our idea was to use a needle in a sheath to reach the ligament. Then a micro-screw would come out of the sheath to enable the surgeon to engage the ligament in a more controlled, safer fashion.

Implement

Implement is the third and final phase of the biodesign innovation process. This is when innovators define the approach that they will use to bring their new solution into patient care. It includes two stages: strategy development and business planning.

A detailed description of these activities is beyond the scope of this chapter. However, the importance of these activities cannot be underestimated. Strategy development and business planning work closely together and should ultimately be integrated into a cohesive approach for getting the new technology to market. Innovators need to carefully define and execute their implementation plan in order to increase the likelihood of the new solution eventually reaching the market.

Strategy Development

Strategy development includes a number of key elements illustrated in the strategy development Fig. 7.2. Defining a comprehensive approach to each one requires expert involvement from consultants or new members added to the project team. A few key considerations in each area are outlined below:

- **Intellectual Property (IP) Strategy** – During concept screening, the innovators determine if a concept is patentable and will have freedom to operate. Now, they develop a more comprehensive approach for protecting the invention. This typically begins with securing an IP attorney and filing a provisional patent application. Then the innovators work with their attorney to think longer-term about a portfolio of utility patent filings for the technology. Patents may be defensive (blocking competitors for the space) or offensive (developing intellectual property in a competitor's area to create different types of barriers). Domestic and international filing should also be considered. A patent portfolio is often the most crucial asset of any medtech start-up, and a strong IP position will often constitute its most important barrier to entry.

Fig. 7.2 strategy development

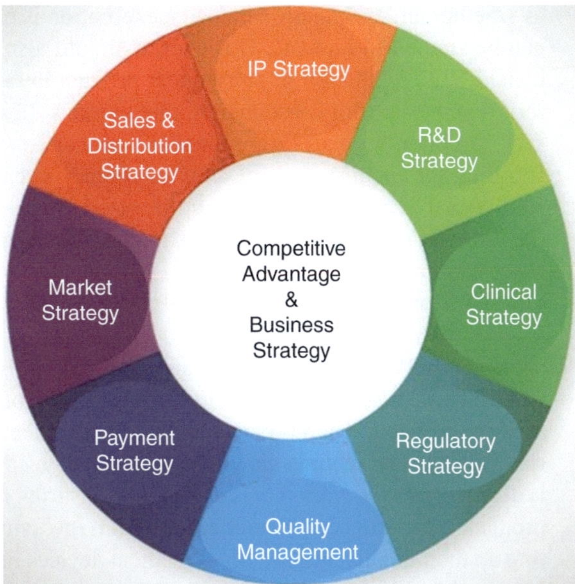

- **Research & Development (R&D) Strategy** – R&D involves defining the scope of work, resources, and approach required to fully develop a safe and effective finished product. Every R&D strategy is iterative, beginning with simple models used to retire key technical risks through bench testing or simulated use testing, and then transitioning to more advanced models used for animal testing and eventually human testing and clinical trials. It also takes into account important considerations such as what will be required to manufacture the technology at scale and the ultimate cost of doing so.
- **Clinical Strategy** – Traditionally, the primary goal of the clinical strategy was to define what clinical evidence was required to demonstrate the safety and effectiveness of the device for regulatory approval, and then outline a plan to accumulate that data. This is still essential, but today increasing amounts of clinical data are also required to justify reimbursement, marketing, and other adoption-related factors. While important, innovators should keep in mind that these secondary outcomes often increase trial complexity, prolong completion time, and increase costs necessary to execute the trials. For this reason, they should work closely with experts in clinical studies to determine the optimal timing, sequence, and design for their clinical efforts.
- **Regulatory Strategy** – From the analysis performed during concept screening, innovators should have a preliminary understanding of how the new technology will be classified based on its risk to patients and the basic requirement of its most likely regulatory pathway. However, as the device is further developed, innovators should work with a regulatory expert to plan and execute a more robust regulatory strategy. Such a strategy will address the immediate requirements of gaining access to the initial target market, including such factors such

as whether an investigational device exemption is required before a new device can be studied in humans. However, it should also take a longer-term view to consider the regulation of subsequent product iterations, as well as the regulatory requirements of subsequent target markets. In some cases, the steps necessary to obtain regulatory approval in one country may be leveraged towards fulfilling the requirements of another country's regulatory body. For example, European CE marking trials may be used for regulatory approvals in other countries if the trials also adhere to the necessary requirements within that other country.

- **Quality Management** – The quality management plan is intended to ensure that the new technology consistently and reliably meets all safety and effectiveness specifications at scale. There are multiple subcomponents of a quality management system, which include: design controls; corrective and preventive actions; production and process controls; equipment and facility controls; material controls; and records, documents and change controls. Quality management is detailed, precise work that is essential to ensuring the long-term viability of the product. Innovators can benefit greatly from involving a quality expert when setting up their quality system. Most medical devices in the US are regulated by the US Food and Drug Administration's Quality System Regulation (QSR) and/or the International Organization for Standardization's ISO 13485 (used voluntarily in the US or as standard in European and other countries).

- **Reimbursement Strategy** – At its most basic, reimbursement strategy involves understanding of the current reimbursement coding landscape to determine if the device will be paid for by public and/or private payers under an established reimbursement code, or whether a new code will have to be secured. It also addresses how local or national coverage will be obtained and at what payment level the technology will be reimbursed.

- **Marketing Strategy** – Defining an effective marketing strategy is focused on better understanding the priorities of key stakeholders and developing compelling product-specific value propositions to convince them to adopt the new technology. Once again, because value propositions are likely to depend on clinical evidence to support them, marketing strategy should be closely integrated with the clinical strategy. The marketing strategy also defines specifically how the product will be priced, positioned (relative to competing solutions), and promoted. With new medical technologies, this often includes the involvement of professional societies and expert physicians (known as key opinion leaders) to help stimulate interest and adoption.

- **Sales & Distribution Strategy** – New technologies can be sold and distributed in multiple ways, including indirect, direct, and hybrid models. The model chosen depends on the company's target customer(s), structure and business model, the product's selling price, and the resources necessary to reach the customer. Indirect models, where a distributor with established customer relationships is chosen to "represent" the product, are often a good choice for lower-cost technologies that do not require a great deal of specialized training. Direct models, where the company sets up its own sales force, can be a good match for higher-cost products that require specialized sales and training support. Each model has different pros and cons (as well as costs) that should be considered carefully before making a decision.

Business Planning

Business planning involves the integration and execution of the strategies developed as part of the previous stage of the biodesign innovation process. The four main business planning activities are described briefly below.

- **Operating Plan & Financial Model** – The operating plan is the mechanism through which the innovators integrate all of the key activities required to take the technology from proof of concept into patient care. It should include and align the key milestones from the R&D, clinical, regulatory, quality, reimbursement, marketing, and sales and distributions strategies. The financial model is then built on the operating plan to determine resources and funding requirements needed to implement the product. It is made up of multiple components as shown in the table below:

Components of financial model	Brief descriptions
Operating plan	High level overview of timing and milestones to take the technology from proof of concept into patient care
Staffing plan	An overview of the personnel needed to execute on the operating plan over time
Market model	Market estimates based on research and assumptions (top-down or bottom-up approach)
Cost projections	Estimated costs of the business, including developing and manufacturing the product, as well as operating the business
Cash flow statement	The actual, usable cash needs of the business
Income statement	A summary of revenue, manufacturing costs, operating margin, operating expenses, and operating income

- **Strategy Integration and Communication** – Once the operating plan and financial model have been developed, innovators can think about how to communicate the needs of the project to attract the required funding, as well as talent and other resources. They should develop a "pitch" that communicates the story of the technology and how it will deliver value to investors and other supporters.
- **Funding Approaches** – Innovators must also determine the appropriate approach to funding the development and commercialization of the technology. Funding may involve a sequential combination of sources, including equity, debt, and/or grants.
- **Commercialization Pathway** – Sometimes innovators will decide to launch a start-up company to bring their new product into patient care. In other cases, they may choose alternate pathways, such as licensing, partnering, or selling the

technology to a corporation. Some inventions are not well-suited to sustain a standalone business and alternate options should be considered. These alternative pathways may be of particular interest to physician innovators who wish to sustain their clinical practice rather than become entrepreneurs.

Case Study: Implement Phase
InSite Medical

To help develop their screw-like device "to more accurately and safely deliver epidural anesthesia in patients requiring pain management to reduce complications," Dr. Wall and his team decided to pursue a start-up company and founded InSite Medical. They applied for and were awarded a government grant to demonstrate the feasibility of the technology and they raised a small amount of seed funding from a group of investors to further develop and test the device.

With regard to their implementation approach, they decided on a regulatory strategy that would make Europe their first market, given the more moderate clinical requirements to receive a CE mark for the technology at the time. For their clinical strategy, they focused on demonstrating a reduction in epidural complication rates with the device compared to the current standard of care. They completed 100+ cases in South America and Europe to support their CE mark submission. Reimbursement for epidural anesthesia was relatively low, and the device itself would be more expensive than current options. However, they hoped to build a positive overall value proposition based on the improved safety profile and lower complication rates associated with the device.

After the company initiated its preliminary market launch in Europe, they encountered some unanticipated usability issues that affected the accuracy of gaining epidural access. As Dr. Wall explained:

> The feeling of a needle hitting the bone as you're pushing it forward is a lot different than a screw hitting a bone. When a screw hits the bone, it's a much more subtle feel. But a lot of physicians relied on the needle hitting the bone and being able to bounce around until they found the epidural space. This approach creates some additional risk, but it works for a lot of people. For them, the screw didn't provide enough feedback to get them to switch positions until they found the epidural space. So, our technology actually made it harder for some users to deliver the epidural quickly and accurately.

The device did improve the safety of epidural placement, however, as the team talked with more and more physicians, they discovered that the target users of the technology did not view safety as a significant concern. They were far more motivated by the usability of the device. According to Dr. Wall, "They told us 'I want to be able to place the epidural quickly and reliably, and then move on to my next procedure.' They didn't want to struggle with an approach that took more time due to patient comfort issues, but also because they got paid by the procedure." The team conducted many user interviews as part of their initial stakeholder analysis, but Dr. Wall acknowledged that they may not have been direct enough with their questions to get truly objective feedback. "Had we listened better to our users earlier, we probably would have realized that they were more worried about the accuracy issue," he said. "But when you ask about safety, everyone tells you it's important even if they have more pressing concerns." He continued, "I think as first-time entrepreneurs we were a little naïve. Everyone wants to be positive when you're asking for their input. And we wanted to listen to the positives, even though that ended up creating problems for us later in the project."

As the usability challenge became increasingly problematic, the company investigated ways to alter the device to include a guidance system to assist with the speed and accuracy of epidural placement. They also considered providing more training to users to help them overcome the usability concern. However, as a small start-up with limited funding, they were not able to raise enough additional investment to pursue either option. This eventually led the team to shut down the company.

When asked what advice he would offer to other aspiring innovators, Dr. Wall went back to the beginning of the project. "Our need statement included two problems – safety and accuracy – and we didn't either listen well enough or do enough research early-on to understand the right one to address. Safety ended up being the more easily solvable problem, so that's the one we ended up going after. But it didn't address the real, higher priority need of the users."

He also recommended seeking more user feedback at all stages of the project and finding ways to get people to be brutally honest when offering their input. "Ask questions that allow users to be critical, and get comfortable hearing negative feedback. In fact, you should fixate on any negative feedback and really make sure you validate and address it as you take your solution forward rather than focusing on the positives, which is the natural and comfortable thing to do."

Even though this particular project didn't work out, Dr. Wall underscored how much he learned from the Insite Medical experience. "Failing doesn't feel great at the time, but it ultimately makes you stronger and better at what you do," he said. "When you fail, take the time to really understand what went wrong. And then bring those lessons to your next project." Dr. Wall has since gone on to co-found additional companies and to advise other innovation projects.

Teaching Biodesign to Physician Innovators

Physician innovators have several different ways they can learn more about the biodesign innovation process. First, they can apply for programs that teach the approach. While Stanford was the first to offer biodesign training, many other universities and organizations across the US and around the world now offer programs based on the same need-driven innovation model. Second, they can seek out resources such as the *Biodesign* textbook [2] and open-source video library [3] to learn and practice the approach themselves. Third, they can explore the many other resources, including peer reviewed articles [4–9], on innovation/entrepreneurship that are currently available (Biodesign is one of many methodologies that can be used).

For those interested in the Stanford Biodesign program, more information is included in the section below.

Stanford Biodesign Innovation Fellowship

The Stanford Biodesign Innovation Fellowship[10] is the most in-depth, comprehensive training program available at Stanford on the biodesign innovation process. It is targeted at post-graduate physicians, engineers, and business people, and requires a full-time commitment from August through June.

The fellows spend the first 4–5 weeks of the fellowship in a structured and fast-paced "bootcamp". It is used as a break-in period to introduce innovators to the biodesign innovation process. Teams of four fellows are formed and presented with a previously selected observation (in the form of a clinical vignette). They use this example to learn and practice the three phases of the biodesign innovation process in a highly accelerated fashion. This provides high-level exposure to what will come when the group begins with their own projects during the remaining 9 months of the fellowship. The bootcamp experience is augmented with didactic instruction and expert coaching to enhance the learning experience.

Identify Phase during Fellowship

The identify phase kicks off with clinical immersion in the assigned clinical area (a different medical specialty is chosen each year). Clinical immersion should occur in multiple venues that span the cycle of care. For example, teams focusing on nephrology-based needs might observe in wards, clinics, dialysis units, homes, post-op units after dialysis access procedures, operating rooms for kidney transplant, ultrasound suites for kidney biopsy, pathology labs for reviewing biopsies, or medical school anatomy labs or microbiology labs. Observations are recorded and translated to preliminary need statements. Then, they are researched and screened against one another to choose the top opportunities. Need criteria are defined to guide the top projects going forward.

Invent Phase during Fellowship

During the invent phase of the Stanford Biodesign Innovation Fellowship, brainstorming includes all members of a team but also may involve additional members, such as content experts in engineering, medicine, or other fields. Concepts are evaluated against the need criteria. Those that show promise are then screened and rescreened objectively in the areas of IP, regulation, reimbursement, business model, and technical feasibility. Concepts with the greatest risks are retired until a lead concept is chosen.

Implement Phase during Fellowship

During the implement phase, the fellows meet with a series of industry experts and consultants. These mentors help the fellows define comprehensive strategies related to R&D, clinical, regulatory, quality management, reimbursement, marketing, and sales and distribution. They also provide guidance on developing the operating model and financial plan, defining a funding approach, determining a commercialization pathway, and ultimately creating a compelling pitch.

Throughout this process, the fellows continue to interact with key stakeholders in their need area – including patients, physicians, representatives of provider organizations, and payers – to stay closely in tune with their needs and priorities.

Life after the Stanford Biodesign Innovation Fellowship

Individuals from various backgrounds participate in the Biodesign Innovation Fellowship. Physician innovators have made up about 36% of the fellows over the last 18 years. Physicians who take part in the program part way through residency, often return to complete their residency training. This may be done during planned surgical research years or during post-doctoral research years within a residency or fellowship program. Some physicians begin Biodesign at the completion of their medical training and others obtain more training in subspecialties after the innovation fellowship year. The largest group of physician alumni chose to pursue an academic career, while others have gone to private practice and/or embraced a start-up leadership path. Some are involved in small or large companies on a full-time or part-time basis. Their roles include chief executive, technical or medical officer, advisor, innovation lead, or board member. Others pursue roles within venture capital firms or incubators. They might also dedicate some time as university adjunct faculty or volunteers.

Academic careers, either in research or clinical tracks, may have variable levels of involvement in innovation or teaching at the university. For example, Stanford Biodesign's fellowship director and other center faculty are Biodesign Innovation Fellowship alumni from various medical specialties; they maintain their academic clinical practice and are members of the school of medicine. They also provide an integral role in the teaching and mentoring of current Biodesign fellows through the fellowship program and lead some of the Biodesign courses at the university. Finally, many are involved in start-ups as advisors or founders.

Fundamentally, training in the biodesign innovation process enables physician innovators to become active contributors in the innovation ecosystem where they can potentially help patients on a significantly larger scale through health technology.

References

1. Kelley T. The art of innovation. In: HarperCollinsBusiness; 2001.
2. Biodesign. The process of innovating medical technologies: Cambridge University Press; 2015.
3. http://ebiodesign.org/.
4. Brinton TJ, et al. Outcomes from a postgraduate biomedical technology innovation training program: the first 12 years of Stanford biodesign. Ann Biomed Eng. 2013;41:1803–10.
5. Steinberger JD, et al. Needs-based innovation in interventional radiology: the biodesign process. Tech Vasc Interv Radiol. 2017;20:84–9.
6. Wall J, et al. The impact of postgraduate health technology innovation training: outcomes of the Stanford biodesign fellowship. Ann Biomed Eng. 2017;45:1163–71.
7. Wall J, Wynne E, Krummel T. Biodesign process and culture to enable pediatric medical technology innovation. Semin Pediatr Surg. 2015;24:102–6.
8. Wynne EK, Krummel TM. Innovation within a university setting. Surgery. 2016;160:1427–31.
9. Nimgaonkar A, Yock PG, Brinton TJ, Krummel T, Pasricha PJ. Gastroenterology and biodesign: contributing to the future of our specialty. Gastroenterology. 2013;144:258–62.
10. http://biodesign.stanford.edu/programs/fellowships.html.

Chapter 8
The Shared Investment Model: Partnering a Venture Capital Fund with a Health System

Monica Jain and Bruce L. Gewertz

Introduction

Necessity drives change in medicine – the need for lower mortality rates, the need for enhanced recovery from procedures, and the need for greater efficiency and value. The urgency for change is further intensified by today's challenging economic environment; hospitals and, especially academic health systems, are under increasing pressure to generate greater financial returns to sustain their multiple missions. Disruptive innovation holds the promise of rapid improvement in all these metrics. That said, the introduction of innovative therapies and devices must always be weighed against the commitment to provide reliable and well-tested treatments.

By definition, disruptive innovations bypass simple modifications of "tried and true" techniques. As a consequence, disruptive innovations are often produced by outsiders or relative newcomers to the fields, who are unburdened by tradition or long-standing commitment to the "old ways." [1] The business setting for disruptive innovation is also different from more incremental improvement processes. Healthcare startup companies rely on leading-edge technologies, often too-untested to attract investment from established companies or standard granting agencies. Since most of these nascent companies fail, the environment is extremely competitive and time sensitive.

M. Jain
Department of Surgery, University of California, San Francisco, San Francisco, CA, USA
e-mail: Monica.Jain@ucsf.edu

B. L. Gewertz (✉)
Department of Surgery, Interventional Services at Cedars-Sinai Health System,
Los Angeles, CA, USA
e-mail: Bruce.Gewertz@cshs.org

© Springer Nature Switzerland AG 2019
M. S. Cohen, L. Kao (eds.), *Success in Academic Surgery: Innovation and Entrepreneurship*, Success in Academic Surgery,
https://doi.org/10.1007/978-3-030-18613-5_8

Given the long odds and intense effort that is required, why should health systems, already burdened by resource intense missions in patient care and research, enter this highly competitive industry? Our hypothesis is that the very survival of academic health systems depends on rapid implementation of fully effective and lower cost care especially for patients with complex illnesses. The irony is that these meaningful advances can only be achieved with close collaboration with individuals not commonly found on medical campuses. In this chapter, we will argue that that a shared investment model is a very effective way to access such entrepreneurs and visionaries. Further, such models allow the cost of investment to be shared with venture capitalists and industry, thereby leveraging the intellectual capital of medical centers and universities.

In a 2016 article, Potter and Wesslund support this argument with three compelling reasons that corporate venture activities are attractive to large health care systems. [2] First, it improves the rapidity of response to market disruption. In today's market, patients and payors alike demand the most effective treatments. Second, exposure to new and radical ideas fosters a culture of innovation among the highly creative population of staff and faculty who do not face the same quarterly financial measures as those in the for-profit world. Third, it creates leverage for academic medicine overall as it is very common for health care groups to invest in concert. This magnifies the impact of the investment while reducing the financial exposure from failure of any given start-up.

Rationale for Creation of a Venture Capital Fund

Too often, bio-medical product development gets quite far along before there is much input from the healthcare professionals who will actually be using these products. The primary goal of industry-health system partnerships is to remedy this shortcoming and more rapidly and efficiently translate ideas into viable products for clinical use. Partnering with venture capital and/or private equity funds allows health systems to directly drive product evolution such that the technology more perfectly fits their own specific needs and structure. As well, when relevant healthcare professionals are involved in product design and development, the last and most critical step of deployment into clinical practice is greatly facilitated by their sense of ownership. As well stated by Nina Nashif of Healthbox, "introducing change in a healthcare delivery system is 20 percent about the technology and 80 percent about the implementation." [2] Most importantly, with early access to state-of-the-art technologies, health systems can provide the highest quality care to their patients.

From the perspective of the entrepreneur, partnering with a health system has many benefits. At the minimum, startups can take advantage of a built-in customer base. Above all else, however, startup companies strongly linked to physicians, nurses, staff, administrators and patients have easy access to a wealth of knowledge and mentorship. Entrepreneurs can rigorously test their products working with the very people who will use them. This offers unparalleled development opportunities and allows for rapid iterations toward a final design.

Basic Models of Shared Investment

In the least complicated version of the shared investment model, the academic institution provides funds to assist in product development by inventors who form separate start-up companies. The principals may originate within the institution or come from outside. To encourage engagement and properly incentivise the inventors, the institution gets a modest equity share. If development is promising, the health system can promote commercialization through further direct investments into those companies and products which best align with its mission. These subsequent investments increase the institutions equity share.

This simple investment model is a variation of the first attempts of Universities, nearly 100 years ago, to profit from the technologies developed within their walls. Perhaps the best example of the early "tech transfer" strategies was the Wisconsin Alumni Research Foundation (WARF) at the University of Wisconsin [3]. This entity was formed to protect the patents and intellectual property of University faculty while facilitating the development and commercialization of worthwhile ideas. The principal mechanism of these initial efforts was establishing licensing arrangements with already established companies, rather than creating new companies based on single products or new technologies.

More substantive and collaborative investment models have increased dramatically in the last decade. These involve health systems forming their own separate venture funds with or without formal partnerships with outside venture capitalist groups (VC). The development of these arrangements has been fueled by the involvement of leading academic institutions such as the Mayo Clinic, Cleveland Clinic, and Partners (Boston) along with other large clinical entities such as Ascension Health (St Louis), Inovo Health (Iowa) and Providence Health (Washington). It is estimated that there are currently more than 50 such funds with individual valuations exceeding $100 million in some cases. Since somewhere near 25% of the total venture capital activity is now in health care, this growing interest by the key consumers of these products is not surprising.

To improve success and further "deal flow," the entities often form some type of associated business development programs which can be configured as short term "accelerators" or more long-term "incubators." In these programs, start-up companies are funded for variable periods of time, 3 months in accelerators and up to 2 years in incubators. To facilitate informal interactions with mentors within the medical center, they are usually housed in proximity to the sponsoring institution. Each sponsor brings their unique strengths to the effort; the healthcare entity provides expertise in patient or physician needs while the VC's support marketing and business plan development and provide counsel regarding long term financing options.

Investment and Return

Since any form of shared investment model requires a substantial capital outlay by the health system, it is essential that leadership sees the value of these partnerships and commits to both the initial investment as well as the follow-on investments invariably needed to take the products to market. Development of new technology from initial discovery to commercialization is obviously high risk and mandates that investors are both patient and accepting of setbacks and, even failure. The rewards of successful investments are considerable and include returns from royalty income or favorable "exits" from the acquisition or public offering of the supported companies.

The passing of the Bayh-Dole Act in 1980 allowed universities, non-profit institutions, and small businesses to maintain ownership of their federally-funded intellectual property. The ensuing financial returns with licensing income and royalties have been remarkable. The annual Association of University Technology Managers (AUTM) Licensing Activity Survey found that between 2012 and 2016, while federal, industrial, and other research funding remained stable, licensing income increased considerably by 13% to almost $3 billion in 2016 [4]. Royalties, cashed-in-equity, lump sums and license fees have also risen exponentially. Overall, research institutions received meaningful equity from almost half of all of the start-ups formed in 2016. In an era of declining reimbursement per unit for clinical work, these alternate activities can provide much needed unrestricted funds for academic support and re-investment.

While non-monetary benefits are less easily quantitated, they are equally important. In our experience as well as that of others, the excitement of these business ventures allows the spirit of innovation to become ingrained in the institution, making very real contributions to the missions of education and research. Contrary to common wisdom, entrepreneurial activity and industry partnerships do not promote a movement away from academic careers and do not adversely effect more fundamental research. A recent study of 6840 science and engineering doctoral students at 39 U.S. universities demonstrated that basic science research activity, the number of publications, and interest in an academic career were not significantly different between labs that encouraged entrepreneurship and labs that did not [5] In addition, labs that encouraged entrepreneurship were more likely to report invention disclosures. Seen this way, it can be argued that a focus on innovation nurtures discovery at all levels, including basic and translational work [6].

Medical innovation also leads directly to numerous other avenues for research funding. The Small Business Innovation Research (SBIR) and Small Business Technology Transfer (STTR) programs of the National Institutes of Health and the National Science Foundation provide additional federal sources of funding for academic departments [7]. Under these programs, small businesses may apply for grants dedicated to technology commercialization. Although universities and other research institutions may not apply for these grants directly, they may be subcontractors to either home-grown or external small businesses who are funded by these grants. Other options for research funding include the numerous federal and private agencies that back technology transfer activities and translational research. The opportunities for industry-based research financing are also substantively enhanced by increased exposure. Finally, the positive publicity from such discoveries can also help attract philanthropic funds to the institution.

Cedars-Sinai Experience

Our experience in venture investment began with the formation of Summation Health Ventures (SHV) in 2014. This $80 million fund included equal capital commitments from Cedars-Sinai and Memorial Care Health Systems. Collectively both non-profits have seven hospitals with >2500 licensed beds and nearly 5000 affiliated doctors.

Our investment strategy was focused on companies that met two requirements: (1) that the two health systems could add value during product development and (2) that we would plan to use the finished product in our operations. Thus our personnel became both contributors and customers. The final rationale for investments is that if it added value for Cedars-Sinai and Memorial Care, it would be attractive to many other hospitals. Hence, the valuation of the companies we invest in would be increased.

SHV largely avoids very early stage companies, concentrating on products that have achieved or will soon achieve FDA approval. Primary areas of interest are new medical devices, non-invasive surgical techniques, and especially information technology to help monitor patients and connect them to their caregivers. The focus is not to hold majority investment positions in the start-ups and we directly encourage other health system funds and major VC's to join in. The investments are generally made during Series A raises rather than seed rounds although we do provide small seed investments, with options to convert to stock, in companies that may develop into more attractive investments.

One of the most critical concerns of any fledgling venture fund, is receiving sufficient leads and contacts to allow a sufficiently rich "deal flow." Over the last 4 years, we have performed initial review of more than 500 potential investments of which about 50 have had some level of due diligence carried out. We assume this high level of activity reflects both the strategic value of our institutions and their personnel, and their potential sales base. A meaningful advantage of our engagement is introductions to our network of partnering VCs and other academic medical centers who can both aide in technology development and become customers.

To date, three of our original investments have returned value much greater than our investment upon their acquisition by larger companies; another 4–5 are poised for sale, Most importantly, a number of these products are adding value right now to our operational efficiency.

Given our positive early experience with Summation Health Ventures, we formed our own accelerator partnering with Techstars, a US-based venture firm that hosts mentorship-driven business development programs in many sectors beyond health care. Techstars mentored companies have enjoyed an enviable record of viability; about 90% of companies who go through their programs are still in business 2 years later, as compared to the base success rate of similar enterprises of 10%.

Every 6 months, a competitive call for interested start-up companies attracts about 500 applications from all over the world. We select 10–12 companies and host them for 90 days on our campus, providing $40,000 per month of support for each. During this intense period of time, Cedars-Sinai clinical and academic personnel mentor the companies, helping to further develop the innovative technologies and integrate them into established care delivery systems. All of the companies in the first two cohorts signed research or commercial contracts with Cedars-Sinai or other academic medical centers. In collaboration with Cedars-Sinai physicians, multiple start-ups performed and published well-controlled studies of their products. Most importantly, the engagement of over 250 physicians, residents, nurses, executives, and other staff in over 1000 h of meetings with the start-ups in this program demonstrates the innovative spirit stimulated by this program. Numerous other programs, including Stanford Biodesign, the University of Michigan, Cleveland Clinic Innovations, and the Johns Hopkins Sibley Innovation Hub, have similar highly successful multi-disciplinary medical innovation programs. [8, 9]

Challenges to Health Care Venture Efforts

As well described by Atkinson in 1994, success in any type of venture fund demands creativity, expertise, and experience [3]. These are, in fact, the key attributes of academic medical centers. Success in investing also requires a fourth attribute - singularity of purpose; many of the investments require 5–10 years to mature. Unfortunately, this long-term focus is often difficult to maintain in large health systems and research universities. A number of factors contribute to this problem including complicated relationships between medical schools and "parent" universities, the capital needs of new affiliated hospitals in rapidly expanding systems and the disruptions associated with too frequent academic leadership changes. These challenges are further intensified by the fundamental tension between "doing good" by helping patients versus generating the highest financial returns.

This tension is invariably present in health care venture efforts because both financial and strategic goals are always in play. While attractive returns are undoubtedly a lure of such investments, most health care funds greatly value the ability to gain a market advantage over competitors through early adoption of disruptive innovations.

Three additional ingredients for success cannot be overlooked. [3]

1. <u>Funds must have capital sufficient to match the aspirations.</u> Without enough money to make prudent "follow-on" investments in later stage financing rounds, health care venture funds can be progressively diluted in equity, greatly lowering their return when the products they helped develop are acquired by large companies or receive substantial funding through an initial public offering (IPO). For this reason most venture funds now exceed $80 million of initial assets. Even this size barely provides a sufficient operating margin for enough analytic personnel to handle the due diligence involved in assessing investment opportunities.

2. <u>Academic aspirations</u> should be largely discounted in investment decisions. This is much harder to do than it appears since the intrinsic value of publication and basic discovery are so deeply ingrained in most of the sponsoring organizations. To succeed in venture investment, support of academic laboratories cannot short change the more mundane but essential tasks undertaken to improve product design and more rapidly commercialize innovations.

3. <u>Collaborations are essential on many levels.</u> Obviously, the process of product development will necessarily involve the entire spectrum of staff and faculty as well as institutional infrastructure such as information technology and laboratory facilities. Equally important, hospital-based venture funds must foster positive relationships with outside, often much larger, venture groups. These connections will greatly advantage later stage funding rounds and enable worthwhile products to be developed well beyond the funding capacity of a single investor.

Conclusion

Creating or partnering with a venture capital fund offers many positives for health systems and academic medical centers. It can speed introduction of new and powerful technologies that enhance the care of patients. It offers the potential for substantial financial returns, adding a new revenue stream that can support academic activities. Finally, it stimulates a passion for discovery and commercialization among employees and faculty. All that said, it is a serious business requiring skill sets and experience not normally within the perview of medical enterprises. Recruitment and retention of personnel with these skills is an absolute requirement for success.

References

1. Christensen CM. The Innovator's dilemma: when new technologies cause great firms to fail: Harvard Business School Press; 1997.
2. Potter MJ, Wesslund R. Provider venture caqpital funds: investing in innovation. Healthc Finan Mgmt Assoc. 2016:51–9.
3. Atkinson SH. University-affiliated venture capital funds. Health Aff. 1994;13:159–75.
4. AUTM U.S. Licensing activity survey: FY2016. Oakbrook Terrace, IL; 2016.

5. Roach M. Encouraging entrepreneurship in university labs: research activities, research outputs, and early doctorate careers. PLoS One. 2017;12(2):e0170444.
6. Sanberg PR, Gharib M, Harker PT, et al. Changing the academic culture: valuing patents and commercialization toward tenure and career advancement. PNAS. 2014;111(18):6542–7.
7. Lee Y. 'Technology Transfer' and the research university: a search for the boundaries of university-industry collaboration. Res Policy. 1996;25(6):843–63.
8. Dyrda L. 58 hospitals with innovation programs—2017. Becker's hospital review. 2017.
9. Cohen MS. Enhancing surgical innovation through a specialized medical school pathway of excellence in innovation and entrepreneurship: lessons learned and opportunities for the future. Surgery. 2017;162(5):989–93.

Chapter 9
Creating an Innovation Environment for Developing and Testing Surgical Devices within an Academic Medical Center

Paul A. Iaizzo and William K. Durfee

History of Innovation in Surgery at the University of Minnesota

Owen H. Wangensteen

For 37 years (1930–1967), Owen H. Wangensteen, MD, chaired the Department of Surgery and was considered the "mentor of a thousand surgeons" who "created the milieu and the opportunities for great achievements by many of his pupils" (Fig. 9.1, Table 9.1) [1]. Dr. Wangensteen encouraged his medical students, residents, and junior faculty to step out of the box, innovate, and solve problems. Based on his strong belief in collaborations, he instituted a two-year surgical PhD program for all residents which was the first of its kind in the country.

Wangensteen himself was a surgical innovator, pioneering advancements in gastrointestinal surgery. He developed a gastric suction device, the "Wangensteen suction", to successfully treat bowel obstruction and an aseptic anastomosis technique for surgeries to remove cancers or ulcers. In 1948, Wangensteen founded the University's Cancer Detection Center. These innovations were optimized by a large number of surgical faculty investigators, an expertise that continues today.

P. A. Iaizzo (✉)
Department of Surgery, Institute for Engineering in Medicine, University of Minnesota, Minneapolis, MN, USA
e-mail: iaizz001@umn.edu

W. K. Durfee
Department of Mechanical Engineering, University of Minnesota, Minneapolis, MN, USA
e-mail: wkdurfee@umn.edu

© Springer Nature Switzerland AG 2019
M. S. Cohen, L. Kao (eds.), *Success in Academic Surgery: Innovation and Entrepreneurship*, Success in Academic Surgery,
https://doi.org/10.1007/978-3-030-18613-5_9

Fig. 9.1 Owen H. Wangensteen served as chair of the Department of Surgery at the University of Minnesota from 1930 to 1967. Source: Historical perspective of cardiovascular devices and techniques associated with the University of Minnesota. In: Iaizzo PA, editor. Handbook of Cardiac Anatomy, Physiology, and Devices, third edition. Springer International Publishing AG, Switzerland, 2015, Fig. 25.2

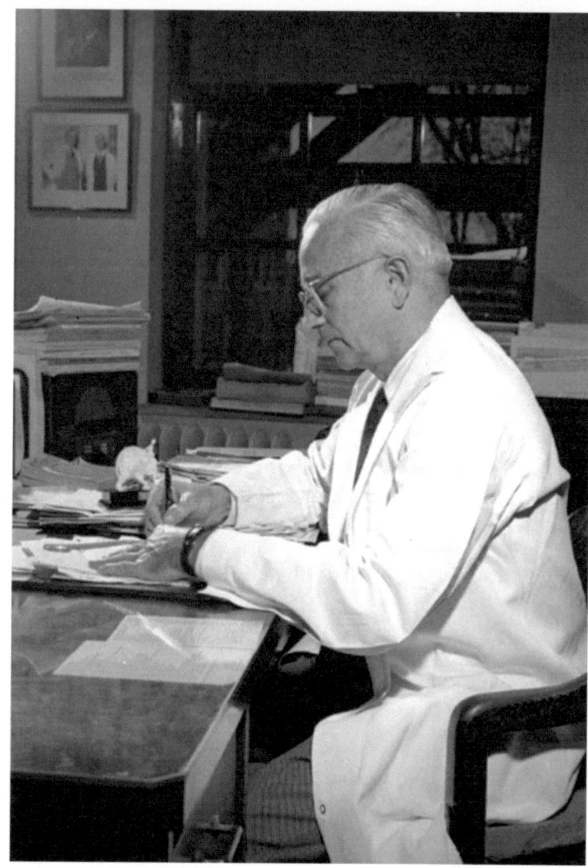

Table 9.1 Department of Surgery at the University of Minnesota: Chairs/Interim Heads

Surgery Department Chair/Interim Head	Position	Years Served
Arthur C. Strachauer	Department Chair	1925, 1927–1929
Owen H. Wangensteen	Department Chair	1930–1967
John S. Najarian	Department Chair	1967–1993
Edward W. Humphrey	Interim Chair	1993–1994
Frank B. Cerra	Interim Chair	1994–1995
David L. Dunn	Department Chair	1995–2005
David A. Rothenberger	Interim Chair	2005–2006
Selwyn M. Vickers	Department Chair	2006–2013
David A. Rothenberger	Department Chair	2013–2016
Sayeed Ikramuddin	Department Chair	2017-present

C. Walton Lillehei

The era from 1950 to 1967 was an incredible time for cardiac innovation within the University of Minnesota's Department of Surgery, in the newly emerging fields of open-heart surgery and medical devices. In the early 1950s, the innovative surge was credited to the fact that many surgical residents returned from World War II, where they had routinely experienced life and death situations when managing patients within surgical field units. Their heart patients were dying and had little chance of survival without the novel techniques that were successfully implemented in Minnesota.

One of these young war-experienced surgeons was C. Walton Lillehei, who returned from leading surgical field units in North Africa and Italy to the University of Minnesota (Fig. 9.2). Lillehei, who completed both MS and PhD degrees at the University of Minnesota, and his team launched many surgical innovations during

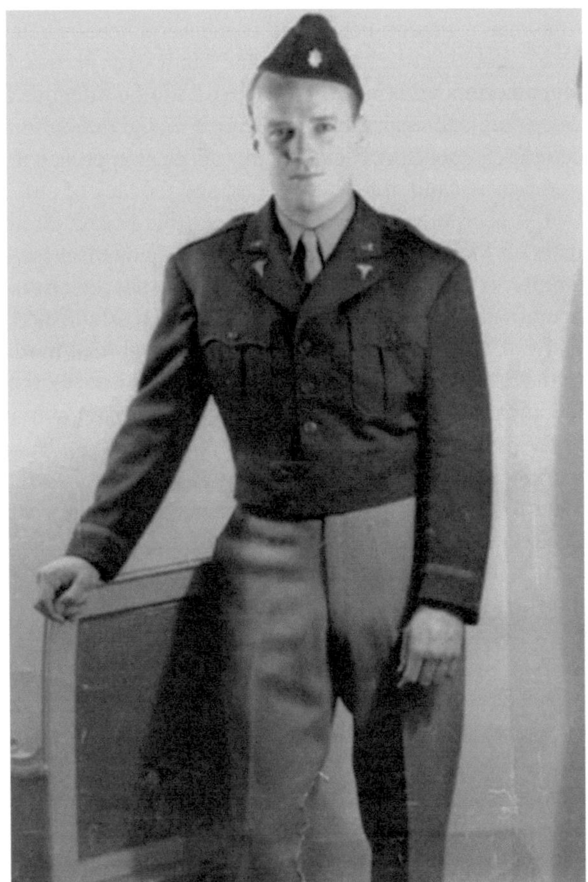

Fig. 9.2 C. Walton Lillehei in army uniform. Source: Historical perspective of cardiovascular devices and techniques associated with the University of Minnesota. In: Iaizzo PA, editor. Handbook of Cardiac Anatomy, Physiology, and Devices, third edition. Springer International Publishing AG, Switzerland, 2015, Fig. 25.3

this period. Their preclinical canine research laboratories were located in the basement of the Mayo Hospital Building, which now houses the Department of Surgery's Visible Heart® Laboratories [2].

Prior to 1950, congenital heart defects were responsible for 1% of all deaths in children. There were no methods for conducting external heart surgery and no techniques to oxygenate the brain during surgery; therefore, only the simplest surgeries could be performed on the beating heart. When the medical profession began to view the heart more physiologically, researchers and clinicians began to develop new ways to repair and replace worn-out parts of the heart. Innovations in the field of cardiac surgery flourished. One of the next major milestones in cardiac surgery was the first open-heart surgery performed using hypothermia, a procedure first attempted on September 2, 1952 by Dr. F. John Lewis and others at the University of Minnesota. This procedure allowed the University of Minnesota team (Drs. F. John Lewis, C. Walton Lillehei, Mansur Taufic, and Richard Varco) to successfully complete a 5½-minute repair of the atrial septum of a five-year-old patient. This was the first time that a surgeon performed intracardiac repair under direct visualization, which was recognized as a significant landmark in the history of cardiac surgery. Hypothermia with inflow stasis proved to be effective for some of the less complicated surgical repairs, but it was not a viable option for more extensive cardiac procedures. Major drawbacks for this surgical approach at that time were the inability to rewarm a cold, nonbeating heart and the lack of clinical defibrillators [3].

Extracorporeal circulation by controlled cross-circulation was introduced clinically on March 26, 1954 at the University of Minnesota after a minimal amount of animal experimentation (Fig. 9.3). The use of cross-circulation for intracardiac operations was an immense departure from established surgical practice at the time and was considered as a major breakthrough that motivated numerous innovations in the area of open-heart surgery [4]. However, the risks to donors included blood incompatibility, infection, air embolism (stroke), and/or blood volume imbalances. Forty-five patients (aged 5 months to 10 years) underwent open-heart surgery with the cross-circulation approach at the University from March 1954 to July 1955. Prior to these pioneering surgeries, such patients were considered to have lesions that were hopelessly unrepairable. Of this group, 22 (49%) of the patients lived to survive more than 30 years and to lead normal productive lives, and 11 of the female long-term survivors subsequently gave birth to a total of 25 children who were free from any congenital heart defects [5].

During this period, an intense competitive but collaborative relationship existed between the University of Minnesota and the Mayo Clinic (Rochester, MN, USA), the only other primary site for open-heart surgery. Lillehei recalled in his interview with G. Wayne Miller (author of *King of Hearts*) how his team would travel to the Mayo Clinic to watch Dr. John Kirklin and his colleagues operate on weekends [6]. Dr. Kirklin was successfully using a modification of the Gibbon heart-lung machine (Fig. 9.4) and, after observing his achievements, Lillehei began a slow transition away from cross-circulation and toward using a heart-lung machine designed by the University. Although its clinical use was short-lived, cross-circulation is still considered today as one of the most important stepping stones in development of the discipline of cardiac surgery.

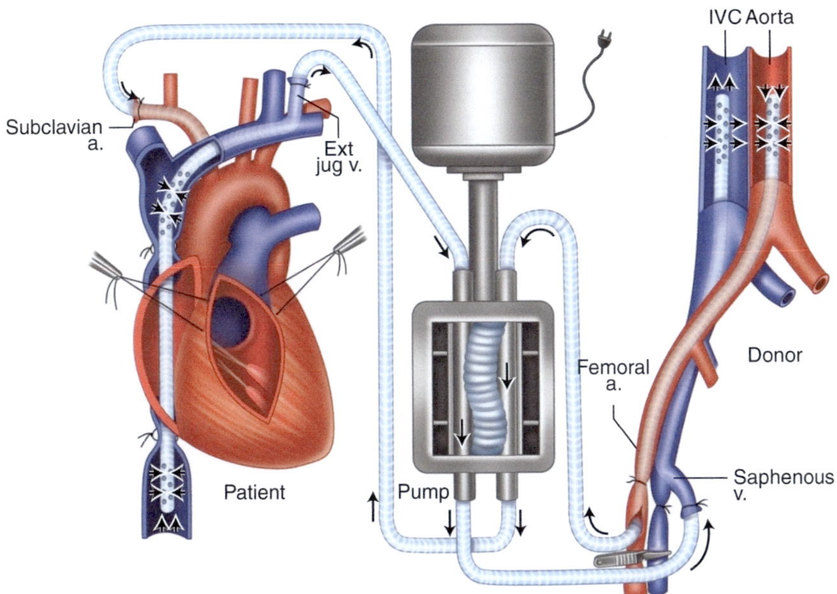

Fig. 9.3 Diagram of cross-circulation. Source: Historical perspective of cardiovascular devices and techniques associated with the University of Minnesota. In: Iaizzo PA, editor. Handbook of Cardiac Anatomy, Physiology, and Devices, third edition. Springer International Publishing AG, Switzerland, 2015, Fig. 25.8

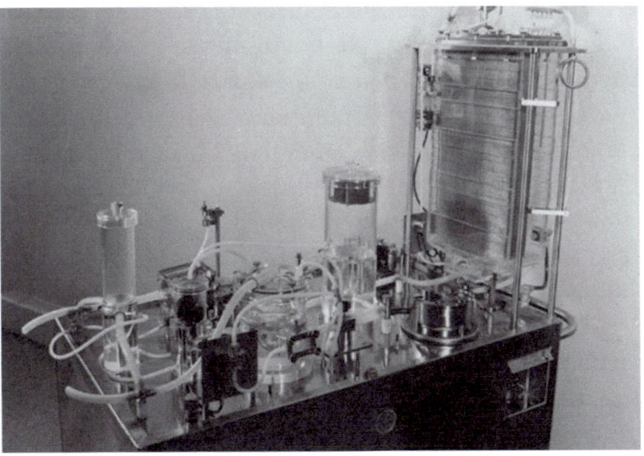

Fig. 9.4 Mayo Clinic's heart-lung machine was the size of a Wurlitzer organ; it cost thousands of dollars and required great skill to operate. Source: Historical perspective of cardiovascular devices and techniques associated with the University of Minnesota. In: Iaizzo PA, editor. Handbook of Cardiac Anatomy, Physiology, and Devices, third edition. Springer International Publishing AG, Switzerland, 2015, Fig. 25.9

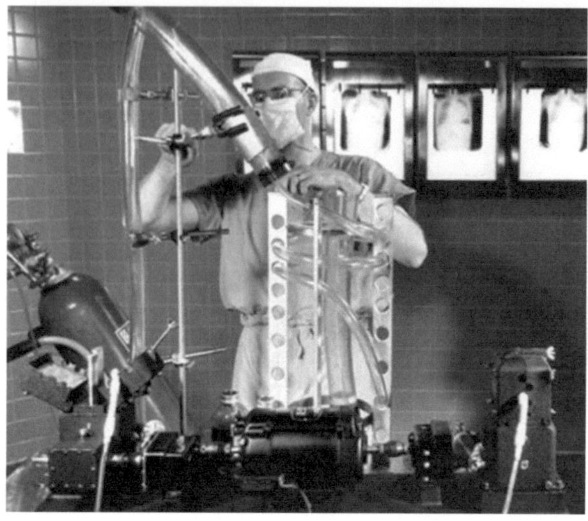

Fig. 9.5 Richard DeWall with his bubble oxygenator in 1955. Source: Historical perspective of cardiovascular devices and techniques associated with the University of Minnesota. In: Iaizzo PA, editor. Handbook of Cardiac Anatomy, Physiology, and Devices, third edition. Springer International Publishing AG, Switzerland, 2015, Fig. 25.10

In the 1950s, Richard DeWall worked at the University of Minnesota as an animal attendant in Lillehei's research laboratory. After being challenged by Lillehei, DeWall brought to fruition a dramatic technological breakthrough in 1955, by developing the first bubble oxygenator with a unique method for removing bubbles from freshly oxygenated blood (Fig. 9.5). Two important components in the Lillehei-DeWall bubble oxygenator were the tubing and silicon antifoam solution. The tubing was Mayon polyethylene tubing (typically used in the dairy and beer industries and specifically in the production of mayonnaise) available from Mayon Plastics, a company whose CEO was a classmate of Lillehei's and a graduate of the University's chemical engineering program. The silicone antifoam solution, Antifoam A, was used to coat the tubing to prevent foaming of the liquids being transported. The oxygenator was wonderfully efficient, and its use in a preclinical experimental animal trial and shortly thereafter in patients did not show detectable effects of residual gas emboli. More importantly, this design eventually led to the development of a plastic, prepackaged, disposable, sterile oxygenator that replaced the expensive stainless steel, labor-intensive screen and film devices. The medical industry began to consider using disposable components for the heart-lung machine. Two years after its introduction, the DeWall-Lillehei bubble oxygenator had been used in 350 open-heart operations at the University of Minnesota. DeWall steadily improved the device through three models that continued to be very simple, disposable, heat-serializable devices that could be built to accommodate only the amount of blood required for each patient and then discarded.

In 1956, another one of Lillehei's residents, Vincent Gott, invented a bubble oxygenator in which DeWall's helix design was flattened and enclosed between two heat-sealed plastic sheets (Fig. 9.6). This sheet bubble oxygenator proved to be the key to widespread acceptance of the device in open-heart surgery, because it was

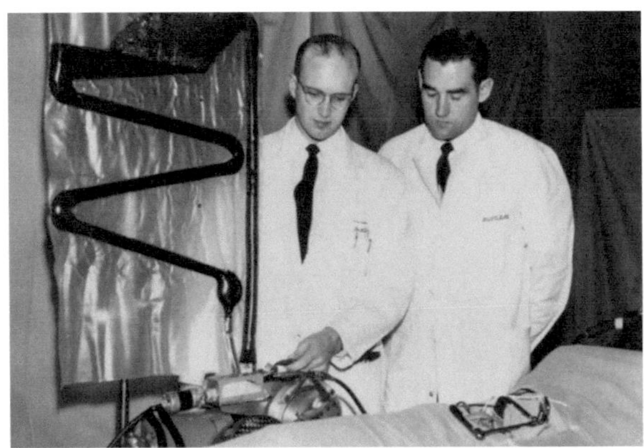

Fig. 9.6 Richard DeWall and Vincent Gott with the first commercially manufactured sterile bubble oxygenator in 1956. Source: Historical perspective of cardiovascular devices and techniques associated with the University of Minnesota. In: Iaizzo PA, editor. Handbook of Cardiac Anatomy, Physiology, and Devices, third edition. Springer International Publishing AG, Switzerland, 2015, Fig. 25.11

inexpensive, disposable, and easily manufactured and distributed in a sterile package. The University of Minnesota eventually licensed the rights to manufacture and sell the device to Travenol, Inc. With the bubble oxygenator and techniques developed by Lillehei and colleagues, the University of Minnesota became even more prominent for making open-heart surgery possible and relatively safe [7].

Heart Block and Development of the Pacemaker

An unexpected clinical consequence of the development of open-heart surgery was the discovery of a revolutionary new concept for treatment of complete heart block. At that time, with the only existing treatment for complete block being positive chronotropic drugs or electrodes applied to the surface of the chest, there were no 30-day survivors. In 1952, Paul Zoll, a Boston cardiologist, invented the first pacemaker, which was a large tabletop external unit with a chest electrode. It was successfully used to resuscitate patients in the hospital, but the transcutaneous delivery of 50–150 volts through the chest was incredibly painful for children and typically left scarring blisters.

Complete heart block developed in 10–20% of Dr. Lillehei's early patients undergoing closure of ventricular septal defects, and hospital mortality was 100% in this group of patients. Early fatality from heart block was completely eliminated with the use of myocardially placed electrodes in combination with an external plug-in electric stimulator [8]. This method of treatment, suggested by Dr. John A. Johnson, a professor of Physiology at the University of Minnesota, required electrical stimuli of small magnitude, provided very effective control of the heart rate, and was nearly painless. However, it required an AC electrical source, limiting

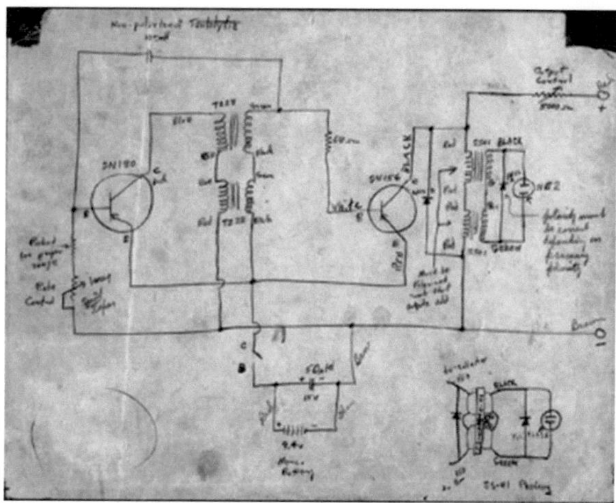

Fig. 9.7 Earl Bakken's original design for the battery-operated pacemaker. Source: Historical perspective of cardiovascular devices and techniques associated with the University of Minnesota. In: Iaizzo PA, editor. Handbook of Cardiac Anatomy, Physiology, and Devices, third edition. Springer International Publishing AG, Switzerland, 2015, Fig. 25.12

patient mobility. It was first used by Dr. Lillehei on a patient on January 30, 1957; subsequently an 89% survival rate for patients with prior heart block was reported. The first pacemaker pulse generator was a Grass Physiological stimulator borrowed from the University's Physiology Department. This procedure was designed for short-term pacing, with removal of the wires 1–2 weeks after the heart regained a consistent rhythm.

Surgical operating rooms in the late 1950s were equipped with EKG and pressure monitoring devices, and the vacuum tubes required frequent monitoring and maintenance to keep them running and calibrated. Hence, the University Hospital subcontracted with a local electric equipment repair company, Medtronic, run by Earl Bakken and his brother-in-law Palmer Hermundslie. Bakken was a trained electrical engineer who received his degree from the University of Minnesota. Following a 1957 storm during which all electrical power service failed in the University Hospital, Lillehei asked Bakken to design a battery backup for their pacemaker system to avoid deaths in heart block patients due to power failures. In 1957, Bakken developed a circuit modified from a diagram for a transistorized metronome described in a *Popular Electronics* magazine (Fig. 9.7). During this period, Bakken spent many hours working in the operating rooms alongside Lillehei, and they became steadfast friends.

On April 14, 1958, the battery-powered, wearable pacemaker was first used clinically. Bakken's transistor pulse generator made a miraculous overnight transition from preclinical animal testing to clinical use. Dr. Vincent Gott successfully demonstrated proof-of-concept of Bakken's first prototype on an animal with an imposed heart block in the Surgery Department's research lab (Fig. 9.8). That night, Lillehei used that same battery-powered pacemaker on a young, critically ill child.

It was this wearable battery-powered invention that set the stage for further development in the cardiac pacing industry. For the next decade or so, it would become common practice to put new devices or prototypes, even fully implantable ones, into clinical use immediately, and then iron out the imperfections later based on accumulated clinical experience. This humanitarian practice developed because most of the

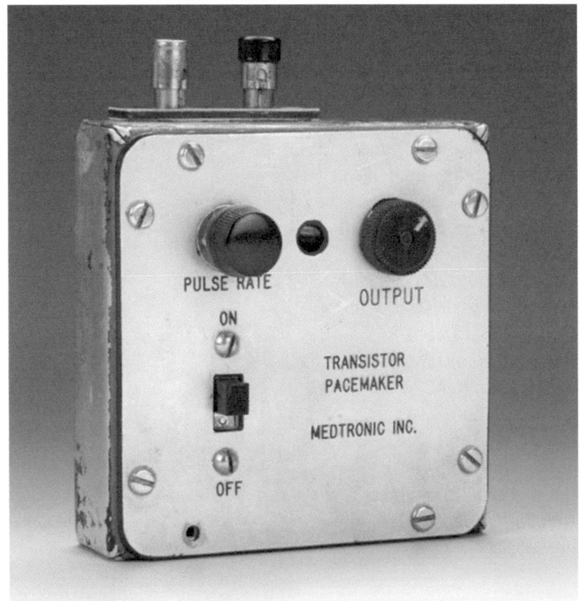

Fig. 9.8 First pacemaker prototype. Source: Historical perspective of cardiovascular devices and techniques associated with the University of Minnesota. In: Iaizzo PA, editor. Handbook of Cardiac Anatomy, Physiology, and Devices, third edition. Springer International Publishing AG, Switzerland, 2015, Fig. 25.13(a)

early patients were close to death, and no other treatments existed [9]. It should be noted that the Food and Drug Administration (FDA) was created by the U.S. government in 1938, but it did not assume the role of regulating medical devices until 1976.

Years later, both Lillehei and Bakken have named Professorships at the University of Minnesota. The current holder of the Bakken Professorship is John Bischof, Director of the Institute for Engineering in Medicine (IEM) at the University. In addition, the Lillehei Heart Institute (LHI) was created in 2002 to honor past accomplishments with the C. Walton Lillehei museum and support the future through its unique research and educational programs [10]. LHI is an interdisciplinary institute within the Academic Health Center and Medical School at the University of Minnesota, made possible by a generous gift from Kaye Lillehei, wife of C. Walton Lillehei.

In December 2007, at a celebration of the 50th anniversary of the wearable battery-powered pacemaker, the University of Minnesota awarded Earl Bakken with an honorary MD degree (Fig. 9.9). In the same month, the University's Department of Surgery hosted the first annual Bakken Surgical Device Symposium to celebrate this legacy. Since its inception, this symposium has focused on topics related to cutting-edge medical devices and promotes the idea of innovation. Dr. Bakken passed away in 2018 at the age of 94, but his legacy will continue to inspire the next generation of medical device developers.

Heart Valves

Initial development of prosthetic heart valves involved the search for biologically compatible materials and hemologically tolerant designs, and early successes could

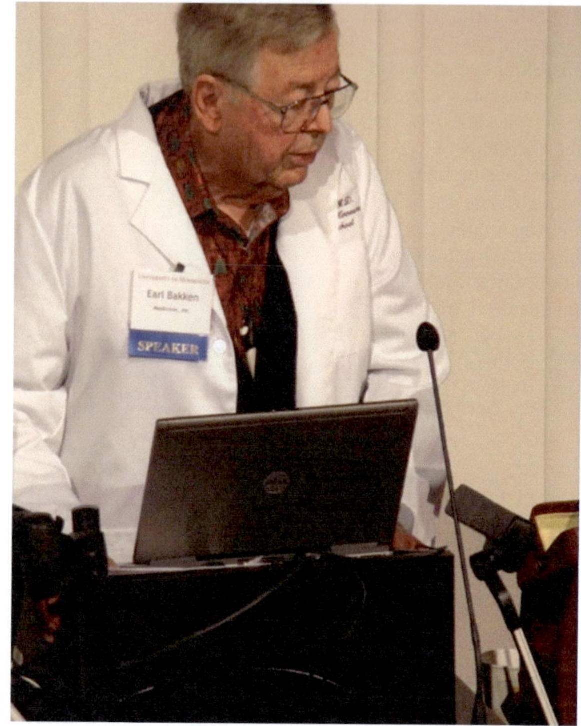

Fig. 9.9 Earl Bakken, founder of Medtronic, received an honorary MD degree from the University of Minnesota in 2007, at the first Bakken Surgical Device Symposium hosted by the Department of Surgery. Source: Historical perspective of cardiovascular devices and techniques associated with the University of Minnesota. In: Iaizzo PA, editor. Handbook of Cardiac Anatomy, Physiology, and Devices, third edition. Springer International Publishing AG, Switzerland, 2015, Fig. 25.15

not have been achieved without the union of these two factors. Initially, as there was no satisfactory mechanism to scientifically achieve these goals, the trial and error method was used, with much of the early work being performed at the University of Minnesota. The development of prosthetic heart valves became the purview of several cardiovascular surgeons who collaborated with engineers. To distinguish one valve from the others, each prosthesis was identified and named after its surgeon-developer [11].

Lillehei and his colleagues developed several different valves: (1) a non-tilting disc valve called the Lillehei-Nakib Toroidal Valve in 1967; (2) two tilting disc valves, the Lillehei-Cruz-Kaster in 1963 and the Lillehei-Kaster in 1970; and (3) a bileaflet valve, and the Lillehei-Kalke in 1965 (Fig. 9.10). The St. Jude bileaflet valve was designed by Chris Posis, an industrial engineer who approached Demetre Nicoloff, MD, a cardiovascular surgeon at the University of Minnesota. This valve had floating hinges located near the central axis of the rigid housing as well as an opening to the outer edge of each leaflet, leaving a small central opening (Fig. 9.11) [11]. Nicoloff first implanted this valve in October 1977, and it provided the foundation for St. Jude Medical to become a significant biomedical device company. Dr. Nicoloff was asked to serve as the medical director of the

Fig. 9.10 The Lillehei-Kalke rigid bileaflet prosthesis (1968). Source: Historical perspective of cardiovascular devices and techniques associated with the University of Minnesota. In: Iaizzo PA, editor. Handbook of Cardiac Anatomy, Physiology, and Devices, third edition. Springer International Publishing AG, Switzerland, 2015, Fig. 25.16

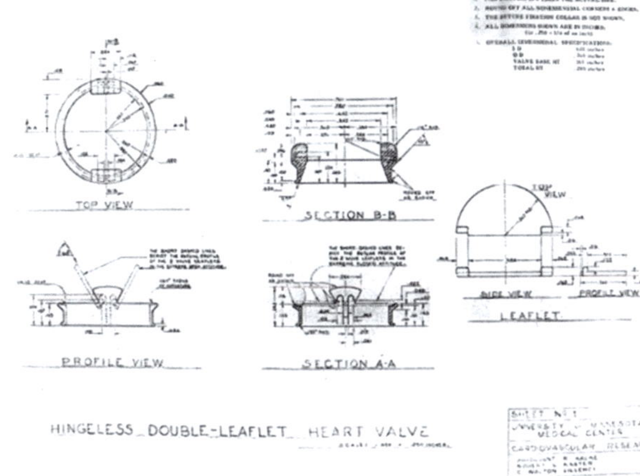

Fig. 9.11 St. Jude bileaflet prosthesis developed in 1976. Source: Historical perspective of cardiovascular devices and techniques associated with the University of Minnesota. In: Iaizzo PA, editor. Handbook of Cardiac Anatomy, Physiology, and Devices, third edition. Springer International Publishing AG, Switzerland, 2015, Fig. 25.17

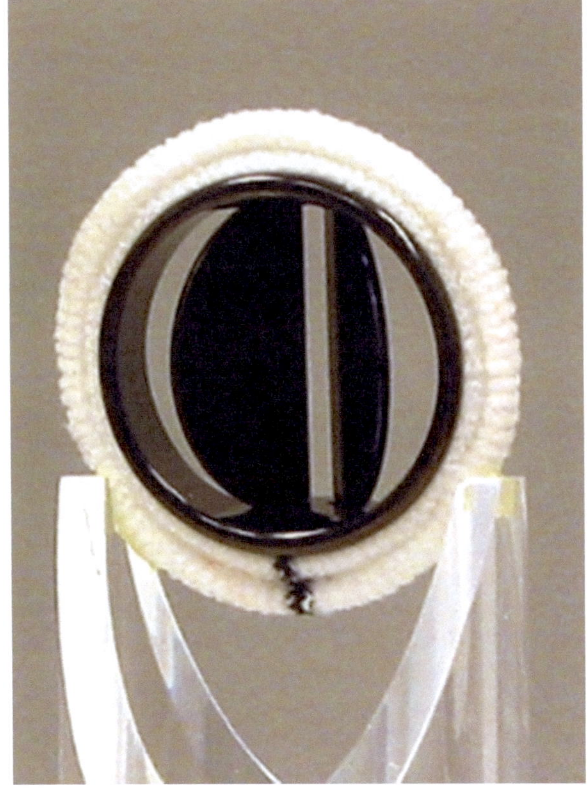

new company, however he declined due to the demands of his clinical practice. Rather, he suggested that Dr. C.W. Lillehei be named as medical director, a post he held until his death in 1999 [11].

Most past and current valve designs were evaluated in animal trials at the University of Minnesota. These trials have been coordinated by Richard Bianco, Director of Experimental Surgical Services, who has more than 35 years of experience at the University working with clinicians, scientists, and engineers on the design, evaluation, and redesign of cardiac valves [12].

John S. Najarian

While surgical innovation in the cardiac area generated better techniques, enhanced surgeons' ability to perform open-heart procedures for longer time periods to enable more complex procedures, and developed new and exciting valves and pacemakers, another branch of surgical innovation at the University of Minnesota focused on organ transplantation. John S. Najarian was appointed professor and chair of the Department of Surgery at the University of Minnesota in 1967, and over time he developed one of the world's largest transplant programs which included numerous milestones: (1) the first pancreas transplant; (2) the first kidney transplant in diabetic patients; (3) the first successful liver transplant; and (4) the first successful bone marrow transplant (Fig. 9.12). Najarian also led the development and manufacturing of antilymphocyte globulin (ALG), a key transplant anti-rejection drug. While eventually exonerated from all charges, Najarian was indicted on several counts related to the sale and use of ALG in 1995, which ended its active use in transplant procedures.

Other Surgical Innovators at the University of Minnesota

In 1969, Richard Varco, Henry Buchwald, Frank Dorman, and Perry L. Blackshear (Mechanical Engineering) invented the implantable drug pump. This device was initially used for the delivery of heparin in 1975, then for the intra-atrial delivery of chemotherapies beginning in 1978, and for administering insulin for patients with diabetes in 1980. Dr. Buchwald is also well recognized as one of the pioneers of bariatric surgery for developing and performing novel gastric bypass techniques (Fig. 9.13a) [13].

Dr. Frank Cerra, a surgical trauma specialist, served as the Department of Surgery chair in 1994–1995 and eventually as the Dean of the Medical School at the University (Fig. 9.13b). He is credited for developing the national model of inter-professional care for patients in need of surgical intensive care, a model that sparked the development of numerous innovative devices, approaches, and procedures [13].

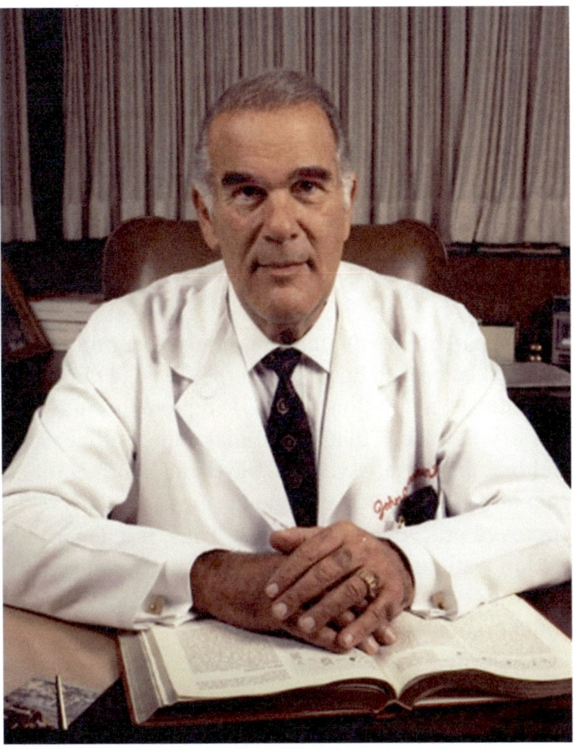

Fig. 9.12 John S. Najarian, chair of the Department of Surgery at the University of Minnesota in 1967, developed one of the world's largest transplant programs. Courtesy of the Department of Surgery (https://www.surgery.umn.edu/about/our-history/najarian-era)

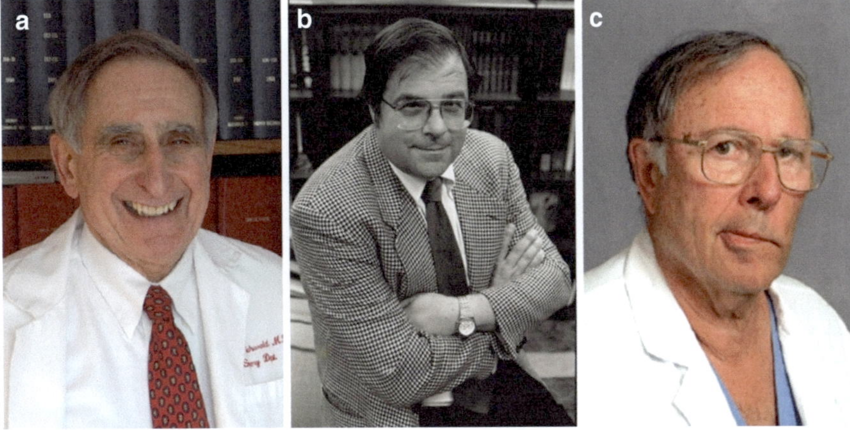

Fig. 9.13 (**a**) Henry Buchwald, (**b**) Frank Cerra, and (**c**) Arnold Leonard

During the 1970s and 1980s within the Department of Surgery, Dr. Arnold S. Leonard spearheaded the implementation of neonatal and pediatric intensive care units, as well as a fly-in service to transport critically ill children. Leonard also developed a double-lumen catheter to improve the intravenous delivery of fluids (Fig. 9.13c) [13].

The University of Minnesota's Innovation Ecosystem and the Institute for Engineering in Medicine

Figure 9.14 shows the medical innovative process in its simplest form. The process can be broken down into three steps: (1) find the problem or need; (2) invent or generate a solution; and (3) implement and test. Most surgeons can easily identify the needs that would make their clinical work easier because they live and breathe these issues and have ideas for solutions. The challenge is that surgeons likely do not have enough time to convert their solutions into clinically approved procedures or devices. Thus, if a department or institution wants clinical innovations to be developed internally, then efforts must be made to create an innovative atmosphere, complete with adequate facilities and a culture of collaboration.

The University of Minnesota is one example of an institution with a strong medical device innovative environment, primarily due to these factors: (1) Minnesota has a strong local medical device industry; (2) the University of Minnesota is a comprehensive land-grant institution with a broad range of departments, faculty, and facilities to foster innovation; (3) The Medical School is within walking distance of the College of Science and Engineering; and (4) various centers and institutes have been created to promote medical innovations, for example the Institute for Engineering in Medicine and the Earl E. Bakken Medical Device Center. In addition, other departments and institutes on campus are part of this innovative environment, e.g., Department of Surgery research labs, Carlson School of Business, College of Design, the 3D Printing Core, and many more. The following sections

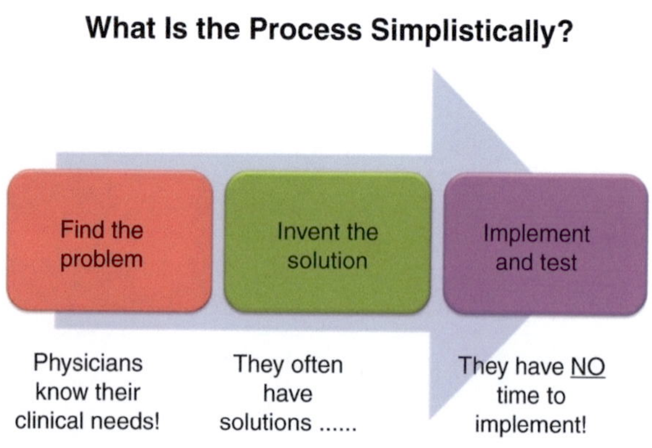

Fig. 9.14 The medical device development process in its simplest form. Physicians know their needs, often have ideas on how to fix them, but have no time to implement them

highlight six entities that are core parts of the University of Minnesota medical innovation ecosystem.

Institute for Engineering in Medicine

The <u>Institute for Engineering in Medicine</u> (IEM) is an interdisciplinary research organization that strives to strengthen collaborative efforts between the disciplines of engineering and biomedicine at the University of Minnesota [14]. Five themes dominate the IEM's research focus: cancer, cardiovascular, medical devices, neural, and regenerative medicine and transplantation. The IEM mission revolves around creating and applying innovative engineering solutions to medical and health problems, in addition to fostering collaborations with industry. To achieve these goals, IEM sponsors three endowed chairs and a fellowship program, as well as various seminars, workshops, and conferences such as the Neuromodulation Symposium, Design of Medical Devices Conference, and IEM Annual Conference & Retreat.

The IEM provides several services to medical researchers around the university. One is the IEM *3D Modeling and Printing Core*. 3D printing is an additive manufacturing method that can build objects directly from a computational model. Unlike traditional manufacturing methods such as milling and molding, 3D printing can construct models of arbitrary complexity relatively quickly. It is a powerful tool for visualizing complex human or animal anatomies, and can be used for surgical planning, physician and patient education, medical procedure training, medical device prototyping, and personalized medical device manufacturing. 3D printing technology is rapidly evolving with advances in materials, resolution, and speed, thus offering greater realism and higher accuracy that in turn enables new medical applications. The 3D Modeling and Printing Core collaborates with medical practitioners and innovators to convert CT or MRI scans of critical anatomy into 3D physical models that can be held and examined to facilitate procedure planning or device design.

The IEM also provides seed funding for interdisciplinary groups seeking to conduct translational research that may lead to future commercialization of novel technologies or procedures. Each year IEM supports a variety of proposal types including the *IEM Group Program* and *IEM Exploratory Grant Program*. Currently, the *IEM Group Program* has provided ~\$60,000 in grants to develop multidisciplinary collaborative research programs from groups of investigators within the Academic Health Center (AHC) and College of Science and Engineering (CSE). These programs are geared to position groups to more successfully secure program/center/group external funding, while supporting significant medical and health research using engineering approaches. The *IEM Exploratory Grant Program* has provided ~\$35,000 to date to support interdisciplinary research projects that explore novel ideas related to medical and engineering research. These proposals involve fundamental or translational science, with a specific hypothesis or deliverable that can produce pilot data to secure external funding or produce intellectual property. These grants pair at least one AHC investigator with a co-investigator from CSE, or vice versa. In order to encourage the development of research across campus, the IEM makes available $6000 in funding for faculty groups to develop collaborations in a focused area. While groups that address research within the IEM's core themes are particularly encouraged, proposals covering new themes are also open for consideration.

Medical Devices Center

The Medical Devices Center (MDC) was established by the University of Minnesota in 2007 [15] and was renamed the Earl E. Bakken Medical Devices Center in 2017. A primary goal of this center is to strengthen interdisciplinary medical device research amongst faculty in the AHC and CSE. The MDC recently opened a new core facility, which includes a computer aided design and precision instrumentation laboratory with 3D printing, an electronic fabrication laboratory, a mechanical prototyping laboratory, a testing room–wet laboratory, an anatomy-physiology SimPortal laboratory, and a multipurpose room for modeling, assembly, demonstrations, and conferences.

The MDC, in collaboration with faculty from the Department of Computer Sciences and various corporate collaborators, has developed a *Virtual Prototyping Lab* with the goal of simulating the placement of existing or novel device concepts within virtual anatomies. Further support is provided by the Minnesota Supercomputing Institute [16], which provides access to high-performance advanced computational resources and user support to facilitate cutting-edge research in all disciplines. Additionally, the institute promotes technology transfer through the interchange of ideas in the field of supercomputing research. Researchers have ready access to informatics, visualization, and application development services.

For early-career individuals who can commit to a year of full-time intensive training in medical technology innovation, fellowship programs offer a unique opportunity. Started by Stanford as part of the Biodesign program, there are now many variations of fellowships offered at universities around the world, including at the University of Minnesota.

At the University of Minnesota, the Earl E. Bakken Medical Devices Center *Innovation Fellows Program* is a full immersion education and product development experience for medical device creation. Now in its 11th year, the fellows program aims to develop the next generation of entrepreneurial and intrapreneurial medical innovation leaders. Each year, eight fellows are selected through a competitive application process. Successful candidates are self-driven and motivated; further they embody an entrepreneurial spirit and have an interest in medical devices. Preferred qualifications are a PhD degree in engineering or science, a medical or health-related degree, a business degree, or substantial industry experience. Typically, a fellowship class includes individuals that represent each of these categories.

The program teaches fellows a disciplined innovation process of understanding clinical environments, finding and screening needs, and developing products and businesses that satisfy those needs. The Phase 1 segment is an eight-week boot camp with intensive didactic lectures drawn from University and local medical technology community experts. Phase 2 of the program consists of 8 weeks of clinical immersion where fellows are integrated into local hospitals and clinics to observe procedures and interact with clinicians. The output of this phase is a set of filtered, significant need statements. Finally, there is Phase 3, product development, which is the bulk of the program during which the fellows, working in small teams and on several projects, ideate and guide concepts through several cycles of build-invent-validate, with the aim of creating new business opportunities that could be further pursued as a startup for entrepreneurs or within an established company for intrapreneurs. As with other fellowship programs, several medical device startups have emerged, surely an indication of the effectiveness of this type of experiential education.

The Visible Heart® Laboratories

The Visible Heart® Laboratories are a unique place to perform translational systems physiology research which ranges from cellular and tissue studies to organ and whole-body investigations [2]. The Visible Heart® labs embody a creative atmosphere, energized by some of the best and brightest students at the University and a lab staff with over 100 years of collective research experience.

Implantable cardiac devices are required to operate within extremely challenging environments. For example, in a typical lifespan of >15 years, a device implanted within a human heart will be subjected to deformations imposed by ~600 million cycles, within a wide variety of anatomies. In most cases, these therapies will in turn induce a positive reverse remodeling of a heart already altered due to disease. Thus, it is important that novel therapeutic concepts are rigorously tested before entering the product development process, to mitigate unforeseen risks. To ensure that these cardiac devices perform safely and as designed when implanted, the industry is highly regulated and design processes have become both lengthy and expensive.

The pre- and post-evaluations of implantable cardiac devices require innovative and critical testing in all phases of the design process. For over two decades, the Visible Heart® labs have utilized a number of research approaches to gain novel insights into the variability of human cardiac anatomies (normal or diseased) as well as the device-tissue interface. To accomplish this, lab faculty and staff employ: (1) an in vitro isolated heart model known as the Visible Heart® which utilizes patented methodologies (US 7045279, DE69922985 T2, and EP1123000 B1); (2) an extensive library of perfusion-fixed human hearts (currently >400 specimens); and/or (3) multimodal imaging in various experimental settings [17, 18]. The use of these methodologies has allowed for detailed examination of device–tissue interactions as a means to evaluate cardiac device placement and subsequent hemodynamic function. The labs routinely coordinate reanimation of hearts on the Visible Heart® apparatus [19]. In such cases, the first several hours of study are dedicated to collecting multimodal images of functional anatomies. Subsequently, or if hearts or heart/lung blocs are not reanimated, specimens are perfusion fixed for future anatomical and educational studies. Internal computed tomography (CT) and magnetic resonance (MR) imaging of the fixed organs are then obtained and presented on the free-access Atlas of Human Cardiac Anatomy website [20]. In addition, almost all specimens on the website are available for in-person examination and measurement at the University of Minnesota; note that some specimens are plastinized.

Experimental Surgical Services

Experimental Surgical Services (ESS) is dedicated to advancing medical technology through translational research. As an integral part of the University of Minnesota's Academic Health Center, ESS is dedicated to educating Minnesota's future healthcare professionals and specializes in research and evaluation of pre-clinical medical devices and surgical techniques [12].

ESS is the birthplace of open-heart surgery. Since that first procedure over 60 years ago, the faculty and staff of ESS have worked to carry on the tradition of performing the highest quality research to meet the ever-changing needs of patients.

Schulze Diabetes Institute

The mission of the Schulze Diabetes Institute is to develop a cure for Type 1 diabetes [21]. In 1974, the institute developed the world's first safe, effective, and minimally invasive cure using islet transplantation. Due in large part to successive improvement of these protocols, human islet transplantation to reverse Type 1 diabetes now matches the success rate of whole organ pancreas transplants. The institute coordinates a robust clinical trials program, and is one of only nine facilities in the U.S. selected by the NIH to conduct Phase III clinical trials, the final round of studies before the FDA decides whether to approve islet transplantation as a standard therapy for Type 1 diabetes.

Basic and Translational Laboratories in the Department of Surgery

The Division of Basic & Translational Research is an intellectually diverse group of nonclinical Department of Surgery specialists that represent a wide-ranging skill set. Areas of expertise include laboratory administration, grant coordination, study design and scholarly manuscript editing. This service is essential to effective basic and translational research studies.

Engaging the Surgical Faculty into Innovation

Membership into IEM

A simple way for surgical faculty to be engaged in innovation is to become an IEM member, which opens significant opportunities to collaborate with colleagues in different disciplines on the development of a new device or procedure.

Clinical Immersion for Nonclinicians

Needs finding is the critical first step in the medical device innovation process, and it is widely recognized that immersion in the clinic is an essential part of educating and/or reeducating the device designer who is not a clinician. Almost all medical device education programs include a period when participants immerse themselves in the clinic which, broadly interpreted, can include procedure suites, operating rooms, hybrid operating rooms, imaging centers, patient rooms, waiting areas, outpatient facilities, assisted living centers, nursing homes, or any other healthcare setting.

For example, the IEM at the University of Minnesota offers a clinical immersion program for nonclinicians, targeted at professionals in medical technology companies who may never have observed a live procedure that uses the category of technology they are developing [14]. The purpose of the immersion program is for participants to develop an understanding of the environment in which medical devices are used. After completing an immersion experience, it is expected that participants will be able to design devices that better meet the needs of patients and clinicians, and to develop relationships with clinicians that could facilitate future collaborations, including future clinical trials. Participants in the program undertake a 1-day or 1-week course and also receive training in a clinical setting on the processes, policies, and procedures related to a range of healthcare situations. Because the course takes place in the clinics at the University of Minnesota hospitals, groups are kept small so they do not interfere with normal clinic operations. This has the added advantage of maximizing the learning experience for students. Participants are charged a fee, with the majority of course revenues distributed to the clinical specialties hosting the program as partial compensation for their time. Some of the services also use the revenue to support their resident research programs.

One of the weeklong clinical immersion programs offered by the IEM focuses on general surgery. Enrolled students include medical device design engineers, quality control individuals, clinical trial and regulatory specialists, marketing professionals, product line managers, and senior executives. The week draws upon many of the specialties in the Department of Surgery at the University of Minnesota, and includes observations of procedures, guidance by residents, participation at pre- and post-surgical rounds and grand rounds, and tours of relevant research and surgical services laboratories. The program is intensive, lasting five full days from 6:30 am to 4:00 pm or later. Surgeries observed might include cardiothoracic, colon and rectal, gastrointestinal and bariatric, pediatric, pediatric cardiac, plastic and reconstructive, surgical oncology, and transplantation. Participants are trained in operating room policies, procedures, and etiquette, including scrubbing in for surgery. Mid-day, students attend lunch and a Q&A session with surgical residents, where they discuss the case they just observed and preview the case for the following day. The experience is structured to encourage participants to observe and study many types of surgeries, because the skilled innovator may be able to connect the dots and leverage their learning in one surgical specialty to invent an innovative device for another specialty.

New Product Design and Business Development Course

While some courses in medical device innovation have an engineering design focus and others emphasize business development, a few universities have developed courses that combine both elements. One example is the graduate-level, two-semester New Product Design and Business Development (NPDBD) course offered by CSE and the Carlson School of Management at the University of Minnesota [22]. For more than 20 years, this multidisciplinary and experiential course has actively engaged students in the product development and entrepreneurial process.

The aim of the course is to educate graduate students in the knowledge and skills required to commercialize a new product, including new medical devices. A secondary aim is to return value to the client company by moving their new product closer to launch. The learning objectives for students include the ability to work with engineering or science specialists and business management teams, the ability to define and achieve both short- and long-term technical and business goals, an understanding of the steps necessary to produce a viable product, and an appreciation for the difference between a plan on paper and the reality of a rapidly evolving technical product market.

The client company sponsors a team of engineering and business students to work for 9 months (over two semesters) on a specific product. Drawing upon guidance from their client, faculty coaches and industry advisors, the student teams conduct background research and then develop a working prototype and an accompanying business plan, which the client carries forward to launch.

Each project addresses market feasibility (What is the need? Do customers want the product?), technical feasibility (How do we design, prototype, and manufacture the product?), and financial feasibility (How much money would the company make?). The overall NPDBD process has four steps:

1. **Discover**: Understand the context and explore the opportunity space
2. **Define**: Define the customer need and state the problem

3. **Create**: Create a solution to the need
4. **Deliver**: Deliver on the solution

Each year, the course hosts six or seven projects, with a mix of clients ranging from established large companies to entrepreneurs who have a product idea that might turn into a startup. Large companies pay a fee of $25,000 and small companies $10,000. The NPDBD course has sponsored dozens of projects over its history; see Table 9.2 for a list of projects over the past 5 years.

Because the company sponsors have an interest in controlling the flow of information about the project and in determining who has ownership of new ideas, all students and faculty in the course sign non-disclosure and intellectual property agreements with each of the sponsoring clients. The non-disclosure agreement enables the client to share confidential information with the student team, and the

Table 9.2 Sponsors and Projects of the New Product Design and Business Development Course, University of Minnesota (2012–2017)

Year	Sponsor	Student Team Project
2016–2017	IKC America	Product to treat veterinary injuries
	Spinal Designs	Product to alleviate back pain
	Agora Investment	New type of backpack
	SelfEco	Self-fertilizing planter for coffee beans
	3VO Medical	Birthing aid
	Medtronic	Device for treating arterial lesions
2015–2016	Medtronic	Device for transcatheter heart valve
	Medtronic	Sensor for cardiac ablation procedures
	Agora Investment	New inline skate concept
	Digital Design Studios	New way to treat bunions
	IKC America	Product to treat athletic injuries
	University of Minnesota	New toothbrush
2014–2015	Medtronic	Product for transcatheter aortic valve replacement
	Medtronic	Method to access heart for cath lab procedures
	Borkon	Product related to womens' health
	Shooting Lab	Product for training basketball shooting skills
	YOXO	New toy using recycled materials
	CCEFP	New applications for small hydraulics
2013–2014	Medtronic	Monitoring system for cryoablation
	EmbraSure Medical	New way to tie the jaw shut
	Tactile Medical	Active compression garment
	Boread Medical Tech.	Femoral artery access device
	Modiron	Method for removing wrinkles from clothing
	Medical Devices Center	Monitoring anesthesia motor block
2012–2013	GeneSegues	Skin patch for drug delivery
	Gromit & Bronk	Child stroller
	Medical Devices Center	Ablation monitoring system
	Medtronic	iPad product information app
	Smiths Medical	Warming blanket
	Smiths Medical	Vascular access
	Surgical Robotics Lab	Surgical skills testing system

For complete project list, see www.npdbd.umn.edu
CCEFP Center for Compact and Efficient Fluid Power

intellectual property agreement assigns patent ownership to the client for any inventions created by the students or faculty.

In addition to team meetings and meetings with the client company, the course includes didactic lectures that cover the basics of the product development process. For example, students receive instruction in sketching, low-resolution prototyping, and patent searching, as well as how to define and research markets, how to gather primary market data through voice-of-the-customer observations and interviews, and how to financially value a new product or business.

Design of Medical Device Conference

The lifelong student of medical device innovation should regularly attend scientific, engineering, and clinical conferences that focus on aspects of medical devices and the medical device design process. For example, the Design of Medical Devices conferences in Minnesota, Europe, and China have offered sessions on device innovation [23]. The following list represents just a small sample of other conferences that provide sessions on innovation:

- Transcatheter Cardiovascular Therapeutics (TCT)
- International Conference for Innovations in Cardiovascular Systems (ICI)
- Catheter Interventions in Congenital and Structural Heart Disease (CSI)
- Heart Rhythm Society (HRS)
- European Society of Cardiology (ESC)
- MedTech Conference (AdvaMed)
- International Engineering in Medicine and Biology Conference (IEEE EMBC)
- Biomedical Engineering Society Annual Meeting (BMES)

Resident Researchers

Although the Department of Surgery at the University of Minnesota does not require their surgeons to pursue a PhD degree, they recommend that residents take one or 2 years within their training program to perform basic or applied research. This work is usually completed under the tutelage of a faculty member that oversees ongoing research programs.

Training the Next Generation of Surgical Innovators

Books and handbooks are excellent resources for students of medical device innovation. While there are many textbooks on product and engineering design, a more modest selection is available with a focus on medical technology innovation and development. Some of the more popular texts include:

- Medical Device Innovation Handbook (WK Durfee and PA Iaizzo)
- Biodesign: the Process of Innovating Medical Technologies (P Yock, S Zenios, J Makower, T Brinton, U Kumar, J Watkins, L Denend, T Krummel, and C Kurihara)
- Medical Instrumentation: Application and Design (JG Webster)
- Design of Biomedical Devices and Systems (PH King, RC Fries, and AT Johnson)
- Contextual Inquiry for Medical Device Design (MB Privitera)
- Medical Device Design (P Ogrodnik)

The medical instrumentation text by Webster [24] has long been used in biomedical engineering instrumentation and electronics courses, but does not cover the innovation process. The short text by Privitera [25] is a detailed description of needs finding via observations and interviews, but is restricted to that portion of the innovation process. The King book [26] provides complete coverage of the engineering design process of medical devices, with less coverage on finding needs or developing a business case for a product. The Ogrodnik text [27] describes most of the medical device design process with an emphasis on what is needed to navigate the regulatory path. The most comprehensive reference is the 952-page *Biodesign* textbook from the Stanford group [28], a step-by-step guide to all aspects of the medical technology innovation process with many case studies. The text follows the *Identify-Invent-Implement* process popularized by the Stanford group, and is one of the few resources that covers the complete process including building a business case for a product. Finally, there is the Medical Device Innovation Handbook published by the Bakken Medical Devices Center at the University of Minnesota [29], which covers much of the same material, but in a more compact format. This handbook originated in the innovation workshops described elsewhere in this chapter, and is available as a no-cost download (z.umn.edu/mdih) for anyone wanting to learn about the medical technology innovation process.

Innovation Workshops

There are also several workshops and short courses sponsored by universities, conferences, and trade organizations, targeting professionals who wish to become medical device innovators. For example, each year the IEM offers two weeklong courses, one in advanced cardiac physiology and anatomy [30] and the other in the anatomy and physiology of the pelvis and urinary system [31]. The cardiac course was specifically developed for cardiovascular device designers and managers, many of whom never studied physiology or anatomy in college or graduate school. The course includes lectures on anatomy, cardiac performance, heart disease, surgical procedures, and cardiac devices, among other topics. The lectures are supplemented with hands-on cadaver gross anatomy labs in which students work in teams to dissect a human heart. Table 9.3 shows a typical schedule for this course. This short course format is an effective way to obtain academic training in a short, intense period.

Table 9.3 Typical Schedule for Advanced Cardiac Physiology and Anatomy Course (University of Minnesota)

Monday		
Welcome	Metzger	7:45 AM
Course introduction/general review of the cardiovascular system	Iaizzo	8:00 AM
Cardiac myocytes	Barnett	9:00 AM
The conduction system of the heart	Iaizzo	10:00 AM
12-lead ECG (Demonstration)	Howard	11:00 AM
LUNCH (provided)		12–1 PM
EKG Lab—Biopac Systems	VHL graduate students	12:30 PM
Control of coronary blood flow during normal and disease states	Katz	1:30 PM
Thoracic surface anatomy and great vessels	Weinhaus	2:30 PM
Gross Anatomy Lab 1: Thoracic surface anatomy, subclavian region and great vessels	Weinhaus/Cook/ Iaizzo	3:00 PM
Keynote Presentation: "Resiliency: Excelling in a Tough Environment" Dr. Rosemary Kelly, Professor and Chief, Division of Cardiothoracic Surgery, University of Minnesota		7:00 PM
Tuesday		
Cardiac development	Martinsen	8:00 AM
Mechanical aspects of cardiac performance: blood pressure, heart tones, and diagnoses	Hutchins	9:00 AM
Large mammalian comparative cardiac anatomy	Hill	10:00 AM
Cardiac energy metabolism	Iles	11:00 AM
LUNCH (provided)		12:00 PM
Use of device-based approaches to treat cardiovascular diseases associated with increased sympathetic activity	Osborn	1:00 PM
Congenital cardiac disease	MacIver	2:00 PM
Surface anatomy of heart and lungs	Weinhaus	3:00 PM
Gross Anatomy Lab 2: Lungs, great vessels and coronary vessels	Weinhaus/Cook/ Iaizzo	3:30 PM
Wednesday		
Catheter ablation of cardiac arrhythmias	Roukoz	8:00 AM
3D electrophysiologic cardiac mapping	Laske	9:00 AM
Pacing and defibrillation	Eggen	10:00 AM
Valve anatomy and transcatheter valves/minimally invasive valve repair procedures	Bateman	11:00 AM
LUNCH (provided)		12–1 PM
Interventional cardiology: stents, closure devices, etc.	Raveendran	1:00 PM
The University of Minnesota: one of the pioneering institutions in the field of cardiovascular surgery	Iaizzo	2:00 PM
Internal anatomy of the heart and posterior mediastinum	Weinhaus	3:00 PM
Gross Anatomy Lab 3: Internal anatomy of the heart and posterior mediastinum	Weinhaus/Cook/ Iaizzo	3:30 PM

Table 9.3 (continued)

Thursday		
Introduction to echocardiography	Sivanandam	8:00 AM
Introduction to anesthesia for cardiac surgery	Loushin	9:00 AM
Monitoring in the ICU	Beilman	10:00 AM
Ex vivo perfusion of the heart or lungs	Huddleston	11:00 AM
LUNCH (provided)		12–1 PM
Clinical anatomy (anatomy review)	Weinhaus	1:00 PM
Gross Anatomy Lab 4: Clinical anatomy (anatomy review)	Weinhaus/Cook	1:30 PM
Small Group Demos: In vitro swine, fresh cadaver	Iaizzo	1:30 PM
Friday		
Experimental gene therapeutics for heart and muscle	Metzger	8:00 AM
Ventricular assist device therapy	John	9:00 AM
Novel visualization of functional human cardiac anatomy employing Visible Heart® methodologies	Iaizzo	10:00 AM
Minimally invasive cardiac surgery: technique overview	Liao	11:00 AM
LUNCH (provided)		12–1 PM
Patient continuum of care following cardiac interventions	Martin	1:00 PM
Cardiac anatomy modeling, virtual reality, virtual prototyping and atlas website tutorial	Bateman	2:00 PM
Gross anatomy lab: Finish dissections and "grand rounds"	Weinhaus/Cook/ Iaizzo	3:00 PM

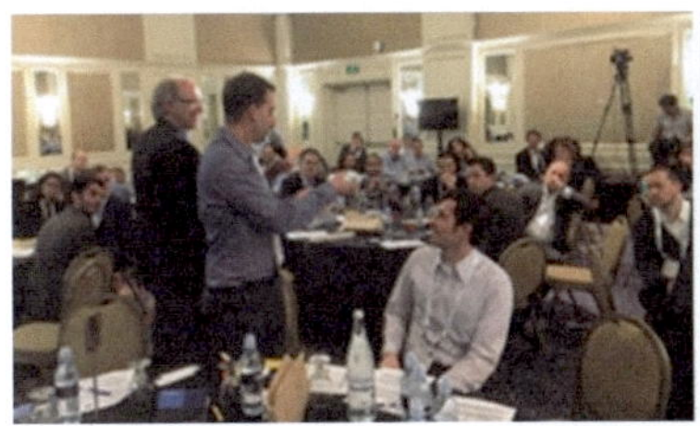
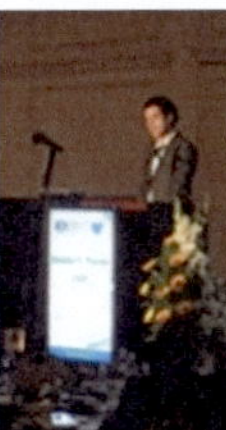
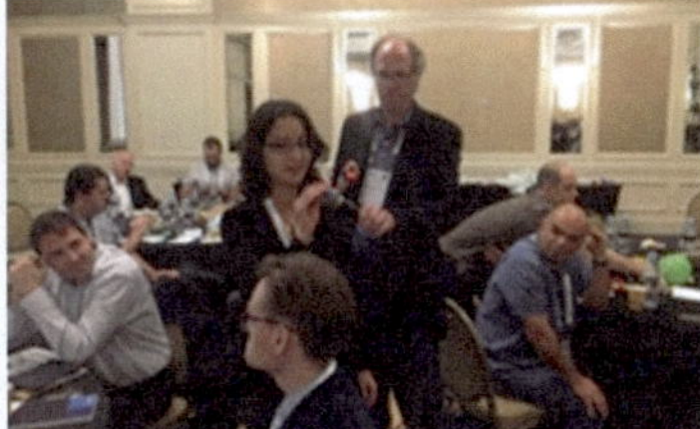

Fig. 9.15 Academy of Innovation at the International Conference for Innovations in Cardiovascular Systems (Tel Aviv)

Other workshops cover the medical device innovation process. One example is the Academy of Innovation, a one-day workshop held in conjunction with the annual International Conference for Innovations (ICI) meeting in Tel Aviv for interventional cardiologists, and targeted to physicians who wish to become entrepreneurs and innovators [32]. The workshop includes three components: (1) didactic lectures on medical technology innovation, including the innovation process, assessing needs, regulatory, patents, and other relevant topics; (2) war stories from seasoned medical technology entrepreneurs to contribute a real-world focus; and (3) hands-on ideation and prototyping so that, by the end of the day, every participant has invented a new medical device concept (Fig. 9.15, Table 9.4).

Table 9.4 Typical Agenda for the Academy of Innovation (one-day workshop on medical technology innovation, part of ICI meeting, Tel Aviv)

08:30–08:50	Reshaping medical pipelines—how clinicians are becoming innovators	Lotan
08:50–09:00	Perspective on innovation development within an Academic Medical Center	Beyar
09:00–09:20	How new medical products are developed—overview of new product development process	Durfee
09:20–09:40	Essentials of creativity—sketching, notebooks, and documenting	Iaizzo & Durfee
09:40–10:00	Brainstorming warmup	Durfee
10:00–10:30	Testing your medical device idea: bench tests, preclinical, clinical trials	Iaizzo
10:30–11:00	Networking break	
11:00–11:45	Innovation exercise 1: Generate ideas	
11:45–12:05	Protecting your intellectual property through patents	Durfee
12:05–12:30	Device innovation: role of regulatory requirements in the U.S.	Oktay
12:30–13:10	Lunch	
13:10–13:30	Inventing, developing, and commercializing new medical devices	Pardo
13:30–13:50	How to determine if a new device is needed—market evaluation and needs assessment methods	Richardson
13:50–14:10	The corporate view of technology assessment and acquisitions	Laske
14:10–14:30	From an idea to exit—the bumpy road today	Essinger
14:30–15:10	Innovation exercise 2: Developing a new cardiovascular product	
15:10–15:30	Digital health revolution—a new player in the innovation market	Fitzgerald
15:30–16:00	Networking break	
16:00–16:20	Team presentations	
16:20–16:40	Fostering a culture of do-it-yourself innovation	Cohn
16:40–17:15	Cardiovascular medical device innovation: a discussion Q&A panel	
17:15	Adjourn	

ICI International Conference for Innovations in Cardiovascular Systems

The hands-on activities are a highlight of the workshop. In one activity, small groups are given a needs statement and asked to prototype a solution to the need, using only the limited supplies provided (paper clip, index card, tongue depressor, foil, clothes pin, and other similar items). The goal is to design a solution for a specific customer-based need and to experience the utility of low-resolution prototyping methods for communicating an idea. In another activity, the group comes up with a need, invents a medical technology that meets the need, and then builds a first prototype using a large "pile of junk," basically parts collected from surgery and procedure suites (catheters, tubes, syringes, valve delivery units, surgical instruments) along with foam board, hot glue, and duct tape.

Summary

Medical device innovation is an exciting and rewarding endeavor and/or career. It requires study, hands-on training, skill, continued lifelong learning, and the ability to bounce back from failures. Innovation within a nurturing environment is a critical parameter for success, with one example being the University of Minnesota. The common advice from experienced entrepreneurs is to: (1) surround yourself with a great team that has knowledge in all associated areas; (2) be passionate about your ideas and champion the technology; (3) fail fast and learn from these failures; (4) plan on working hard; and above all (5) enjoy the process.

References

1. Lillehei CW. The birth of open-heart surgery: then the golden years. Cardiovasc Surg. 1994;B2:308–17.
2. www.vhlab.umn.edu (Visible Heart® Laboratories website). Accessed 19 Dec 18.
3. Lillehei CW, et al. The first open heart repairs of ventricular septal defect, atrioventricular communis, and tetralogy of Fallot using extracorporeal circulation by cross-circulation. Ann Thorac Surg. 1986;41:4–21.
4. Lillehei CW. A personalized history of extracorporeal circulation. Trans Am Soc Artif Internal Organs. 1982;28:5–16.
5. Moller JH, Shumway SJ, Gott VL. The first open-heart repairs using extracorporeal circulation by cross-circulation: a 53-year follow-up. Ann Thorac Surg. 2009;88:1044–6.
6. Miller GW, editor. King of hearts. New York: Crown Publishers; 2000.
7. Moore M. The genesis of Minnesota's medical alley. UMN Medical Foundation Bulletin. Winter 1992.
8. Gott VL. Critical role of physiologist John a. Johnson in the origins of Minnesota's billion dollar pacemaker industry. Ann Thorac Surg. 2007;83:349–53.
9. Rhees D, Jeffrey K. Earl Bakken's little white box: the complex meanings of the first transistorized pacemaker. In: Finn B, editor. Exposing electronics. Amsterdam: Harwood Academic Publishers; 2000.
10. www.lhi.umn.edu (Lillehei Heart Institute website). Accessed 19 Dec 18.
11. DeWall R. Evolution of mechanical heart valves. Ann Thoracic Surg. 2000;69:1612–21.
12. www.surgery.umn.edu/research/research-groups/experimental-surgical-services (Experimental Surgical Services website). Accessed 19 Dec 18.
13. Korostyshevsky D. Cutting edge: the University of Minnesota Department of Surgery 2017 http://z.umn.edu/dosvideo. Accessed 19 Dec 18.
14. www.iem.umn.edu (Institute for Engineering in Medicine website). Accessed 19 Dec 18.
15. www.mdc.umn.edu (Earl E. Bakken Medical Devices Center website). Accessed 19 Dec 18.
16. www.msi.umn.edu (Minnesota Supercomputing Institute website). Accessed 19 Dec 18.
17. Chinchoy E, Soule CL, Houlton AJ, Gallagher WJ, Hjelle MA, Laske TG, et al. Isolated four-chamber working swine heart model. Ann Thorac Surg. 2000;70:1607–14.
18. Hill AJ, Laske TG, Coles JA Jr, Sigg DC, Skadsberg ND, Vincent SA, et al. In vitro studies of human hearts. Ann Thorac Surg. 2005;79:168–77.
19. Iaizzo PA. The visible heart® project and free-access website "atlas of human cardiac anatomy". Europace. 2016;18(Suppl. 4):iv163–72.
20. www.vhlab.umn.edu/atlas (Atlas of Human Cardiac Anatomy website). Accessed 19 Dec 18.
21. www.surgery.umn.edu/research/research-groups/schulze-diabetes-institute (Schulze Diabetes Institute website). Accessed 19 Dec 18.

22. https://carlsonschool.umn.edu/departments/strategic-management-entrepreneurship-department/academic-programs/new-product-design (New Product Design and Business Development webpage). Accessed 19 Dec 18.
23. www.dmd.umn.edu (Design of Medical Devices Conference website). Accessed 19 Dec 18.
24. Webster JG (ed). Medical instrumentation: application and design 4th ed. Wiley, 2009.
25. Privitera MB (ed). Contextual inquiry for medical device design. Academic Press, Waltham MA, 2015.
26. King PH, Fries RC, Johnson AT, editors. Design of biomedical devices and systems. 3rd ed. Boca Raton: CRC Press; 2014.
27. Ogrodnik PJ, editor. Medical device design: innovation from concept to market. London: Academic; 2012.
28. Yock PG, Zenios S, Makower J, Brinton TJ, Kumar UN, Watkins FTJ, Denend L, Krummel TM, Kurihara CQ, editors. Biodesign: the process of innovating medical technologies. 2nd ed. Cambridge: Cambridge University Press; 2015.
29. Durfee W, Iaizzo P (eds). Medical Device Innovation Handbook, 7.0 ed. University of Minnesota Medical Devices Center, 2017. (z.umn.edu/mdih). Accessed 19 Dec 18.
30. www.physiology.umn.edu/degrees-and-programs/industry-professionals/phsl-5510-cardiac-short-course (Advanced Cardiac Physiology and Anatomy Course website). Accessed 19 Dec 18.
31. www.physiology.umn.edu/degrees-and-programs/industry-professionals/phsl-5525-pelvic-short-course (Anatomy and Physiology of the Pelvis and Urinary System Course website). Accessed 19 Dec 18.
32. http://icimeeting.com/academy-of-innovation-day/ (Academy of Innovation/ICI Meeting). Accessed 19 Dec 18.

Chapter 10
Leveraging Multiple Schools into a Multidisciplinary Innovation and Entrepreneurship Program at an Academic Medical Center: The *NUvention* Model

Vineet Sharma, James Sulzer, Michael Marasco, Edward Voboril, Peter McNerney, and Swaminadhan Gnanashanmugam

Introduction

Throughout the course of this textbook, the reader has been introduced to a number of models of fostering medical innovation and entrepreneurship at a variety of academic centers. The Stanford Biodesign model, featuring fellowship teams and a capstone graduate student class, the Cedars-Sinai model involving venture capital funding within a surgical department, the Minnesota model of an innovation center for surgical devices, and the Harvard/Partners in Health model for fostering surgical innovations, have all been featured. This chapter features another model - multiple schools within a university context have been leveraged to create a multidisciplinary, multi-institutional model for medical innovation and entrepreneurship within an academic setting. This model, Northwestern University's NUvention: Medical Innovation, is comprised of a six-month interdisciplinary course, jointly owned and developed by the graduate schools in Engineering, Medicine, Law, and Business. The model features interdisciplinary teams comprised of students from each

V. Sharma · M. Marasco · E. Voboril · P. McNerney
Northwestern University, Evanston, IL, USA
e-mail: vineet.sharma2019@u.northwestern.edu; mmarasco@northwestern.edu; e-voboril@northwestern.edu; peter.mcnerney@kellogg.northwestern.edu

J. Sulzer
University of Texas at Austin, Austin, TX, USA
e-mail: james.sulzer@austin.utexas.edu

S. Gnanashanmugam (✉)
Baylor College of Medicine, Texas Heart Institute, Houston, TX, USA
e-mail: gnanasha@bcm.edu

© Springer Nature Switzerland AG 2019

M. S. Cohen, L. Kao (eds.), *Success in Academic Surgery: Innovation and Entrepreneurship*, Success in Academic Surgery,
https://doi.org/10.1007/978-3-030-18613-5_10

discipline paired with a faculty mentor. Each team is tasked with finding a unique, unmet health care need then leveraging the resources of the various schools, the university, and the greater Chicago area ecosystem to develop a medical device, service or software solution to that need. As part of the process, each team develops a working prototype, an investor presentation and a business plan, which are delivered at the conclusion of the course. The teams are then encouraged to pursue commercialization with support from the entrepreneurship resources at Northwestern and the greater Chicago area. Over the past 11 years since the course's inception, a number of start-up companies and licensed products have arisen out of the course.

In contrast to the other models discussed in this chapter, the idea for NUvention Medical originated with a team of students, an idea that was subsequently supported by key higher level personnel (Sect. 2). The detailed structure and function of the course, highlighting its distinctive attributes, will then be described (Sect. 4). Finally, lessons learned throughout this process will be reviewed (Sect. 5), revealing insights that may have value to the reader looking to start a multi-disciplinary, multi-instutional academic program within their academic institution.

Section 1: Creation of NUvention: Medical Innovation

Setting the Scene: The Northwestern Medical Innovation Landscape Prior to NUvention

Prior to the creation of the NUvention program in 2007, the Northwestern University campus had an underdeveloped entrepreneurship culture, especially within the health care space. However, many of the elements necessary to create an innovation program were present, albeit scattered, throughout the university. On the downtown Chicago campus, Northwestern had top 20 ranked medical and law schools, adjacent to buildings where most of the medical research was being performed. Also next door was the consolidation of the Passavant and Wesley Memorial hospitals, which in 1999 created the $580 M, Northwestern Memorial Hospital Feinberg and Galter Pavillions, a world-class hospital facility, the largest hospital within the city of Chicago.[1]

Within the hospital, numerous world-class clinical departments faciliated successful medical innovators and entrepreneurs. Dr. Nathaniel Soper, vice chair of the department of surgery, was a noted innovator within the field of laparoscopic surgery. He pioneered the adoption of the critical view of safety for laparoscopic cholecystectomy and worked with numerous medical device companies to develop numerous surgical instruments to usher in the era of laparoscopic surgery. Dr. Charles Davidson, chief of interventional cardiology, founded Advanced Stent Technologies in 1998, a company focused on developing stents and delivery sys-

---

[1] https://www.nm.org/about-us/history/northwestern-memorial-hospital-timeline

tems for bifurcated lesions, later acquired by Boston Scientific for \$120 M plus additional contingent payments.[2,3] Finally, in 2005 The Bluhm Cardiovascular institute was created at Northwestern Memorial Hospital with the recruitment of Dr. Patrick McCarthy, chief of cardiothoracic surgery from the Cleveland Clinic and inventor of three different heart valve designs, all licensed to Edwards Lifesciences corporation. The Northwestern downtown campus had talented medical innovators without a cohesive program to unify and leverage those talents and experiences.

Thirteen miles to the north is the university's main campus in Evanston, home to additional outstanding scientific talent as well as top-ranked McCormick School of Engineering and Kellogg School of Management. Northwestern recently enjoyed a successful license of the drug Lyrica/Pregabalin, which netted \$700 M in patent revenues to the university and greatly increased the school's appetite for additional entrepreneurial efforts and opportunities to commercialize its intellectual property.[4] Medical technology start-ups emerged from campus, including Nanosphere, Inc., and Z-KAT (which became Mako Surgical), which enjoyed successful venture rounds and were subsequently acquired.[5,6] However, though there were a few courses involving multiple schools the engineering, business, law and medical school each largely operated within their own silo, with minimal interaction with each other.

Even though there were a number of leading health care institutions in the greater Chicago area there was little interaction between these leaders and the university. Large pharmaceutical and medical device manufacturers including Abbott, Baxter, and Takeda had their headquarters or major offices in the area; large physician associations such as the American Medical Association (AMA) and the American College of Surgeons (ACS) were headquartered in Chicago; Blue Cross & Blue Shield, responsible for insurance coverage for nearly 1/3 of all insured Americans, had its national association's headquarters in Chicago; JCAHO (the joint commission for the accreditation of hospital organizations) had its headquarters in nearby Oakbrook Terrace. However, despite the presence of these large players encompassing various aspects of healthcare, a substantial healthcare start-up scene and culture had yet to materialize, let alone meaningful collaborative efforts between these various entities.

This culture would eventually begin to change on the Northwestern campus, a change that was given a significant boost by the pioneering efforts of a group of students. They conceptualized an interdisciplinary course involving multiple

---

[2] https://www.thestreet.com/story/10013455/1/medinol-competitor-advanced-stent-technologies-secures-30-million-.html

[3] http://news.bostonscientific.com/news-rele, http://news.bostonscientific.com/news-releases?item=58700ases?item=58700

[4] https://research.northwestern.edu/news/legacy-lyrica

[5] https://www.genengnews.com/news/luminex-buys-nanosphere-for-83m/

[6] https://www.wsj.com/articles/stryker-to-acquire-mako-surgical-for-about-165-billion-1380114400

schools to help foster medical innovation and along with passionate faculty members and supportive university leadership, worked to bring this vision into a reality.

An Idea Is Born: "The Life Sciences Innovation Program"

The program that ultimately became *NUvention: Medical Innovation* was conceived in the spring of 2006 by a 2nd- year medical student at Feinberg who was inspired by his experiences as an undergraduate and master's level engineering student during the early years of the Stanford Biodesign program.[7] This student, Swami Gnanashanmugam, had previously worked with Biodesign founder Paul Yock and later with medical device development consulting firms performing venture-capital sponsored research into medical device products. Gnanashanmugam also took numerous early Biodesign courses, including the Stanford Biomedical Technology Innovation two-quarter course, while at Stanford.

When Swami arrived at Northwestern he canvased the other 175 medical students in his class and found that 10–20% had some sort of engineering or industry background, and were interested in working at the interface of medicine and technology and in developing new medical technology. He and a similarly enthusiastic medical student with an industry background, Neel Patel, formed a student group in 2005, called the Life Sciences Technology Club, to develop new ideas into prototype medical devices. However, at Northwestern and in Chicago, the two students found that the infrastructure necessary for medical students to innovate in this space was not yet in place. For example, they could seek out mentors, but there was no formal program for teaching medical students how to innovate medical device technology. And while entrepreneurship courses were available to the Engineering and Business schools, the physical distance between the two campuses posed difficulties in forming interdisciplinary collaborations.

On a trip to Kellogg (Northwestern's Graduate School of Management), they happened upon a newly formed, energetic student group with a similar interest—InNUvation (not to be confused with NUvention). InNUvation was a new student group consisting primarily of graduate students from the Business and Engineering schools, dedicated to increasing student entrepreneurship and innovation. InNUvation's goals were to serve as a hub for entrepreneurship at Northwestern, to enhance the entrepreneurial culture, and to serve students from all Northwestern's schools. InNUvation's co-presidents were Todd Melby, a Kellogg student with an interest in biotechnology, and James Sulzer, a Mechanical Engineering PhD student with an interest in robotic rehabilitation technology. They organized a series of business plan workshops open to all students and created the first university-wide business idea competition, the Northwestern University Venture Challenge (NUVC).

---

[7] https://www.farley.northwestern.edu/we-teach/nuvention/projects/nuvention-medical-history.html

After a series of meetings, the students discussed the idea of modifying the Stanford Biodesign course and fellowship structure to create a novel, hybrid structure that would be ideally suited to Northwestern. They recognized such a course would help unify the substantial resources present in schools of Engineering, Business, Medicine and Law, and the strong healthcare ecosystem in Chicago. Such a course would require coordination and cooperation from the faculty of these schools, as well as clinical faculty from Northwestern Memorial hospital, and would also likely require support from the local healthcare ecosystem, much like the Stanford Biodesign courses. By building such a course, the students would be creating the infrastructure and ecosystem necessary to support innovative device concepts, and helping to foster a culture of entrepreneurship and innovation across the entire campus.

The Initial Prototype: Northwestern's Life Sciences Innovation Program

The students initially named the new creation the "Life Sciences Innovation Program," choosing to name it a program, rather than a course, to emphasize that the new creation was to be more than just a course, but rather a plan or a system within which students would learn how to identify unmet clinical needs, develop solutions to those needs, and gain the skills necessary to achieve the ultimate goal—to commercialize those solutions for the betterment of patient care (Fig. 10.1).

Adapting from the Stanford Biodesign model, of which Gnanashanmugam had first-hand experience, the students sought to create a hybrid that utilized elements of Stanford's fellowship program, as well as its course. In the Stanford program, the primary ethnography was performed by the Biodesign fellows over the span of an initial month or two clinical immersion during the fall. After undergoing a screening

Fig. 10.1 Life Sciences Innovation Program— Cover slide from an early presentation & proposal

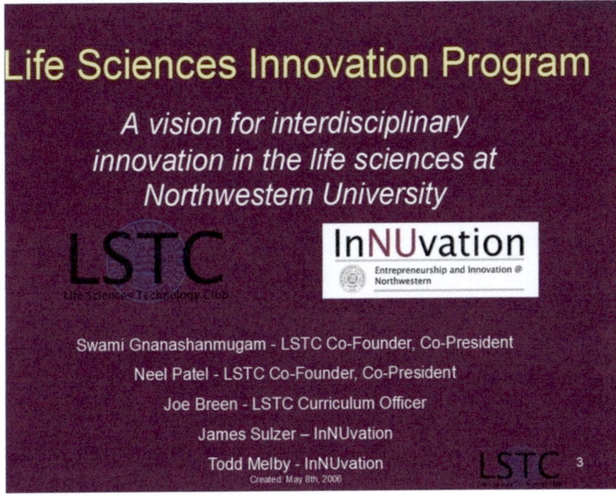

process, left over needs were then offered to students taking the Biodesign course, a 2-quarter, 6-month long course during the winter and spring quarters. Furthermore, clinical immersion by the fellows was typically based on the clinical theme of that year; 1 year might be cardiovascular, the following year might be in orthopedics, and so on, thus, each year, producing needs that typically were clustered around a dominant clinical focus area. Students, predominantly in engineering and medicine, would then adopt these needs, and organically form teams of 4–6 students around a given need of interest, and then undergo the Biodesign process to try to develop a novel, commercially viable solution to these needs. Curriculum would be taught primarily by Professors Yock and Makower, but also relying heavily upon outside guest speakers who were brought in to lend further expertise in relevant areas, such as clinical and regulatory topics, or reimbursement. At the end of the academic year, both fellows and students would present their solutions to a panel of outside experts, who would then judge and critique the solutions. Fellows and students would then decide if they wanted to pursue these solutions further and attempt to make them commercially viable products and companies. Stanford's program was largely funded by outside industry sponsorship, especially for the year long, fully funded fellowship program covering approximately four full-time spots per year. This funding was in large part possible due to connections and relationships forged through successful medical innovation and a track record of entrepreneurship held by Professors Yock and Makower. The program was primarily funded through venture capital and then moved to industry-sponsored educational grants, meaning that it brought funding to the university and thus did not compete for existing resources by being self-sufficient. The Biodesign program thus served as an important predicate case study of interest in terms of campaigning to bring a similar program to Northwestern.

The Northwestern students modified elements of the course and the fellowship to create a hybrid version that differed from the Stanford program to better fit the environment of Northwestern. Rather than focusing on one clinical area per year, the new program would focus on 8–10 clinical areas per year, with a number of areas repeating yearly, and a few clinical areas rotating through every few years. Certain clinical areas that were hotbeds of medical device innovation, such as cardiovascular, orthopedics, GI and general surgery, and interventional radiology, for instance, would be standing clinical areas that would remain permanent every year, whereas other areas such as emergency medicine or otolaryngology would rotate in and out every few years. Each clinical area would have a team comprised of 4–8 students, with at least one student from each of the four graduate schools of law, medicine, engineering, and business, and would involve a lead clinical faculty advisor in that field from Northwestern Memorial Hospital and the medical school faculty. The course would take place in the fall and winter quarters, in a similar 2-quarter, 6-month long format, but it would take place earlier in the year, thus allowing for teams to apply for business plan competitions and other funding resources at the conclusion of the course during the remaining spring quarter. Combining the primary ethnography elements of the fellowship with the course, the teams would be responsible for participating in clinical immersion themselves, coordinated by the aid of the medical students in the course and the clinical faculty lead. Rather than predominantly first year medical students as in the Stanford course, Northwestern Medical students would be fourth and final year medical students, typically paired into their chosen field of interest and study; *i.e.*, a final year medical student interested in general surgery and applying for a general surgery residency would be assigned to the general surgery team. The course would also involve law students, and have a significant didactic focus involving the law school, particularly in the areas of intellectual property, leveraging the expertise of Northwestern's School of Law.

The course would meet formally in a weekly didactic session, the first half of the year taking place downtown where the medical school, law school, and hospital and clinics resided, and taking place in Evanston where the schools of engineering, business, and the prototyping facilities resided, in the second half (Fig. 10.2). During these weekly sessions, held in the evening from 6 pm to 9 pm, the initial hour would feature Northwestern faculty and didactic sessions on a given topic, the second hour would feature an industry or outside speaker to further expound upon the subject, and the final hour would typically be left for team meetings to focus on their project work. Deliverables for the course would include a list of identified unmet clinical needs, a clinical needs screening and assessment, market research, prototype of a medical technology solution or device, an intellectual property assessment, a clinical development and regulatory pathway proposal, a reimbursement analysis, and finally a business plan and final pitch to a group of industry veterans and experts. Funding for the course would include $10 K in prototyping funds to be used by the teams to further develop their solution. The course would culminate in a final presentation or investor pitch to an outside advisory board that would offer their critiques and judgments. The course would be jointly and equally owned by the four schools, and be administered by a committee comprising of faculty members from each school, responsible for their subject area, and a clinical lead faculty member, responsible for recruiting and identifying the clinical advisor for each team, as well an alumni chairperson with significant medical device industry experience to ensure that the course represented as "real-world" an opportunity as possible for the students to learn, identify unmet needs, develop device solutions for those needs, and

Fig. 10.2 NUVention: Medical Innovation Course Planned Structure for 2007–2008

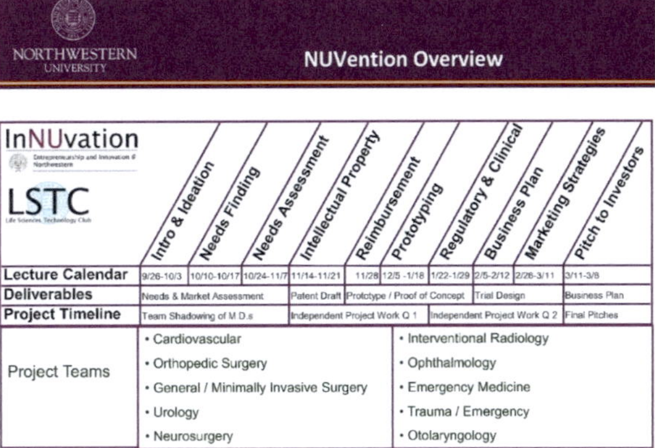

	Intro & Ideation	Needs Finding	Needs Assessment	Intellectual Property	Reimbursement	Prototyping	Regulatory & Clinical	Business Plan	Marketing Strategies	Pitch to Investors
Lecture Calendar	9/26-10/3	10/10-10/17	10/24-11/7	11/14-11/21	11/28	12/5 -1/18	1/22-1/29	2/5-2/12	2/26-3/11	3/11-3/8
Deliverables	Needs & Market Assessment			Patent Draft	Prototype / Proof of Concept			Trial Design		Business Plan
Project Timeline	Team Shadowing of M.D.s			Independent Project Work Q 1			Independent Project Work Q 2			Final Pitches

Project Teams	• Cardiovascular • Orthopedic Surgery • General / Minimally Invasive Surgery • Urology • Neurosurgery	• Interventional Radiology • Ophthalmology • Emergency Medicine • Trauma / Emergency • Otolaryngology

ultimately, if they had so chosen, to try to commercialize those needs in terms of a start-up company. By poising the course to end in the spring, student teams would have more time to decide if they wanted to form a company or otherwise pursue efforts to commercialize their technology.

Those who wished to pursue their plans further had a litany of resources available. Teams could enter their projects into InNUvation's newly created alumni-sponsored business idea competition (NUVC) to gain additional funding for their efforts. Teams would also be introduced to various organizations and agencies both within the university and in the Chicagoland area to help with their commercialization efforts. On-campus groups like the SBOC (small business opportunities center) a law-school group that specialized in helping small businesses with free legal services, and connections to ITEC-Evanston (Illinois Technology and Entrepreneurship Center) and associated grant funding and workspace opportunities would be made available. Futhermore, students could apply for the then recently formed Illinois Biotechnology organization (IBIO) Propel program, an accelerator program sponsored by IBIO to help early stage life science companies by providing entrepreneurs with access to specialized resources and expertise to prepare them for early stage funding, with the aid of grants, awards, business plan competitions, mentorship and networking opportunities.[8]

Students: Grassroots Change Agents

With a plan for the program in place, the students then began a grassroots, bottom-up campaign to try to marshal the resources necessary to bring such a program to the university. The students identified the key elements needed to bring the program to fruition: a.) faculty members from each graduate school who would be interested in teaching and administering the course, and whom could bring in outside speakers to help aid and develop content, b.) clinical faculty members in various disciplines in medicine who would be interested in mentoring student teams and developing novel medical technology innovations, c.) institutional support for the program from administration and leadership within the four schools and hospital, d.) interested, motivated students, who exemplify the phenotype of the entrepreneur and innovator, within the various schools, who'd be interested in taking such a course, e.) an experienced, industry leader or innovator, to ensure that the program stayed true to its mission of ensuring a "real world" like experience for students to undergo the medical technology innovation product development cycle, f.) and finally, a new source of funding, likely external, that would add to the overall university resources, rather than drawing from pre-committed, pre-existing resources. After first recruiting an initial core group and cadre of interested students, the core team of students initially focused their efforts on recruiting faculty, both clinical and academic, to the cause, via a series of individual, one-on-one meetings where they pitched the LSIP

---

[8] http://ibioinstitute.com/propel/

to faculty, garnered their feedback, improved the pitch, and also gauged faculty interest in participating in the course, as well as fit.

In the initial slide presentation, prior to detailing the structure and function of the program, the students initially began by creating a reminder to the faculty and leadership audience of the mission of Northwestern university, both as a whole, and as a function of each of the graduate schools. Focusing on the mission statements, the students articulated the unifying themes—to create leaders, and to contribute to the world by applying knowledge to solve the world's problems (Fig. 10.3).

Over the course of the spring, the students pitched the LSIP concept to approximately 20 members of the faculty from Northwestern's schools of law, business, engineering, and medicine. During the course of these pitches, it was important to reinforce that the program was not meant to compete with existing courses taught by these members of the faculty, but rather to complement them. For instance, if a given engineering course taught rapid prototyping, or a given business school course taught the intricacies of reimbursement, the LSIP course was meant not to replace these course, but rather, to give an opportunity for the learner who had already gone through this coursework and had developed this skill set, to apply the lessons learned and skills gained towards a medical technology innovation project. Furthermore, it provided an opportunity for students to teach other what they had learned in other schools and in other courses, via the framework of the medical technology innovation project. Thus, the course was received as an entity that would complement existing course offerings, rather than compete with them (Fig. 10.4).

In addition, during the course of these presentations, the students ensured that the faculty, students, and leadership who were presented the program were shown in detail how the end product would benefit them, and how the benefits of participating in such an effort would be far greater than the costs of participation (Fig. 10.5). The students showed to each constituent—student, faculty course director, clinical

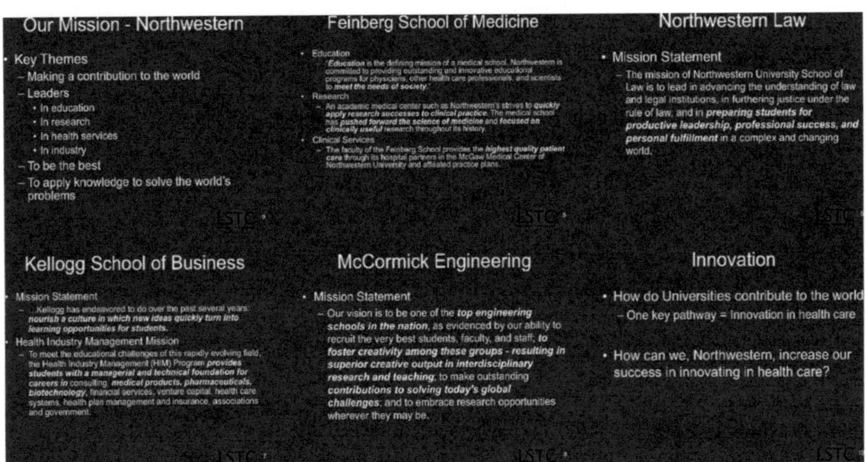

Fig. 10.3 Making a case for innovation—unifying the themes within Northwestern university Graduate schools' mission statements

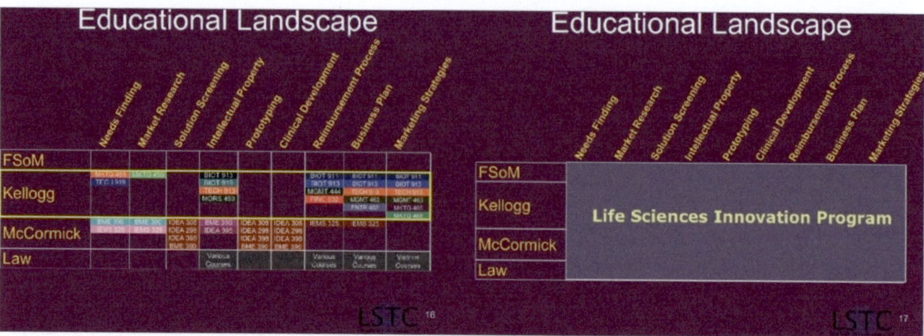

Fig. 10.4 Educational landscape among the four Northwestern graduate schools, circa 2006, highlighting the complimentary nature of the Life Sciences Innovation Program as a course wherein one could apply skills relevant skills gained in other courses to develop a medical technology innovation

Fig. 10.5 What's in it for me—Expectations (costs) vs. benefit for each Nuvention constituent, ensuring that the benefit to each party was greater than the cost

Program Constituents

Participants	Expectation	Benefit
Course Director(s)	• Administer course • Network - invite speakers • Evaluate deliverables & student performance	• Teaching/Course Credit • Research & Publications • Grant Funding • Financial Compensation
Clinical Project Leaders	• Shadowing opportunities • Provide periodic guidance • Evaluate deliverables	• Primary Inventor status • "Free labor" to innovate • Research & Publications
Students	• Highly driven team players • Commitment to innovation • FSOM – participation outside of elective rotation	• Resume builder • Low risk entrepreneurship • "Real world" experience • Professional networking
University	• Support for this initiative • Increasing Incentives for participation	• Interdisciplinary Success • Marketing / Advertising • Product Revenue • Educational Programs

faculty project leaders, and university administrator—how the return on time, energy, and resources for them was ultimately far greater than the investment.

For **Faculty course directors**, expectations included the work of administering the course, creating content our outsourcing course content to experts within their network whom would be asked to present as part of the course speaker series, and to evaluate student deliverables and performance. Benefits included credit for having developed and launched this new initiative, teaching credit or compensation, and being able to participate in any research or publications that arose from the program thereof. For **clinical physicians and surgeons** involved with the team within their sub-specialty area of focus, expectations including providing and coordinating clinical shadowing and immersion opportunities to facilitate the ethnography necessary for finding unmet needs, providing periodic guidance to the teams, and also to help participate in these teams as mentors; benefits included the potential to be part of the primary inventing team, exposure to and access to a talented, multidisciplinary team of students eager to innovate with them in their given field, and of course, the access to participate in the fruits of this combined team labor, be it research, publications, devices, companies, or other efforts. For **students**, a thirst to innovate, the ability to work well in teams, and the commitment to a 6-month course was necessary. Furthermore, for medical students, though the course would involve an initial 4-week immersion, similar to a clinical clerkship, the expectation would be for their active participation for the duration of the course as a contributing team member, for which they would receive an additional 2 weeks, for a grand total of 6 weeks of course credit. Benefits to students included course credit, the opportunity to build their CV or resume via a tangible, medical technology innovation project, an opportunity to experience a life cycle of entrepreneurship and gain "real-world" experience at low-risk, while within a protected academic setting, and network opportunities, let alone the opportunity to potentially develop a solution of their creation into a tangible product or a start-up company. For **university leaders**, support was necessary and vital for success of the program; however, the benefits included a successful, multi-disciplinary, multi-institutional innovation and entrepreneurship program, the ensuing marketing that such a program would produce in terms of raising school stature, the potential to shift culture within the institution to create a more collaborative, innovative, and entrepreneurial environment, the ability to develop closer, stronger ties to industry and potential funding and collaborative opportunities thereof, and of course, the potential for revenue for the university via licensed intellectual property developed through the program.

Over the course of the summer, fall, and winter months, the program was pitched to approximately double that number of clinical faculty members, via the medical students on the core team who encountered various faculty members across multiple different departments during their clinical clerkships. Largely via word of mouth and individual student recruiting efforts, the core group of students spread the word regarding a potential new course offering amongst their classmates, tapping into the latent interest already present, recruiting students who would be interested in taking this course if offered. In this manner, amenable faculty who would be a good fit for the program, both as steering committee leaders, as well as a clinical team leaders, were thus identified and recruited to join the program, as were students, if it were to ever materialize. The excitement building around this new proposed course, from faculty and students alike, ultimately led to introductions with graduate school administration and leadership, and the concept for the course was ultimately presented at the dean and vice-dean level, beginning with the schools of engineering and medicine.

The Importance of Strong Leadership (and Serendipity)

Having thus garnered support and interest from students, academic faculty, and clinical leaders alike, the core group of students progressed to presentations with various vice-deans and deans constituting leadership positions within the schools of engineering and medicine. Of these meetings, by far the most critical and impactful meeting was with Julio Ottino, Dean of the McCormick School of Engineering.

A meeting with the Dean in the summer of 2006 would prove consequential, as Dean Ottino recognized the potential for the new course and its alignment with strategic initiatives he had in mind for the McCormick School of Engineering. A number of critical developments arose from this meeting, including an invitation from the Dean to present the concept for LSIP in the early fall at the strategic planning meeting of the McCormick Advisory Council.

The McCormick advisory council consisted of senior engineering faculty and prominent alumni of Northwestern, and met yearly as part of the strategic planning initiative for the McCormick School of Engineering at Northwestern University. At this meeting, the students had an opportunity to present the concept for the LSIP. Feedback was tremendously supportive. Alumni members of the council demanded that the Dean have the course in place by the following year. Having thus given the dean the mandate to make the program happen, and with the wellspring of support for the initiative from academic faculty, clinical faculty, and students, the pieces soon began to fall in place to make the program a reality.

One such tremendous supporter of the program who met the students initially at the McCormick Advisory Council meeting was Ed Voboril. Ed was a prominent alumnus of Northwestern University, and had enjoyed a successful career in the medical device industry. Most notably, from 1990, he served as CEO of Greatbach Inc., a leading original equipment manufacturer of pacemaker components and electrochemical batteries, named after its founder who invented and developed the very first pacemaker. Voboril heard of the program and at the meeting, met the core student team. He announced that he would be retiring as CEO and Chairman of Wilson Greatbach that year, and heard of the very innovative new program at Northwestern and was interested in being a part of it. In Voboril, the program had its perfect chairperson—an experienced, seasoned medical device industry veteran—who could lend credence and credibility. A fire in his newly constructed home in Arizona cemented Voboril's decision to remain in Chicago and become a new member of McCormick's faculty and as chairperson of the new program, a critical move that would enable the program to become a reality.

Another critical move would soon follow that proved instrumental not only to the formation of LSIP/ NUvention: Medical Innovation, but to the formation of the entire NUvention program and the establishment of the future Farley Center for Entrepreneurship and Innovation. In the summer of 2006, the student leaders piqued the interest of Michael Marasco, at the time an adjunct professor in McCormick, teaching a technical entrepreneurship course for engineers. Marasco was able to work with the students to modify the structure and continue to adapt to the university, soon becoming the leader and driving force behind the program. Dean Ottino appointed Marasco as a clinical professor of Industrial Engineering and Engineering Management in early 2007, with the mandate for making the LSIP program into a reality.

Thus, during the fall of 2006, due to Dean Ottino's leadership and initiative, Voboril was able to formally come on board as the chairperson for LSIP, and Marasco was able to come on board as the Course director from the engineering school, to form the first initial members of the multi-school faculty committee that would be in charge of administering the program. This bold step by the engineering school to make the course a reality had a ripple effect with the other schools, who then quickly followed suit and wanted to become a part of the new initiative.

A transition in leadership at the Feinberg School of Medicine took place, where Dean Lewis Landsberg retired and the new Dean, Larry Jameson, took over. The new Dean immediately saw the benefit of the course, and pledged to make the human resources in terms of faculty, both academic and clinical, available for the program, and committed to support the program. The dean placed vice dean David Johnson on the academic steering committee to be the medical school course director. Dr. Patrick M. McCarthy, one of the first clinical professors contacted about the program and a staunch, enthusiastic supporter from the start, came on board as the clinical faculty course director for the program. Having gotten the approval of the Dean and senior leadership, the students were able to make even further progress with all of their conversations with hospital clinicians and garner further interest in the program. The chairpersons of general surgery, orthopedics, radiology, urology, and all of the clinical departments also agreed to join in in the new and exciting course. Thus, the medical school joined with complete buy-in in the winter of 2006.

With the medical school and engineering school on board, the Kellogg School of Management soon followed. Professor Alicia Loffler, founder of Kellogg's center for biotechnology management, was identified early on in the process as the prime candidate for the Kellogg course director position, and was able to come on board in this capacity officially once the course gained approval by the Dean of the Business school.

Finally, Dean Van Zandt of the law school approved the proposal and appointed Professor Clinton Francis as the course director, one of the first professors contacted in the early pitching process for the course (Fig. 10.6). Professor Francis was a tenured faculty member who taught intellectual property law, intellectual capital management among other areas. Furthermore, he had experience teaching engineers and business students through his involvement in various teaching responsibilities at both campuses, and was able to leverage that expertise as Law school course director.

Given the unique nature of the course, a groundbreaking effort involving four different schools within the university, the core group of students was also incorporated into the steering committee as student directors of the course (Fig. 10.7). As students, having been in the system at each school, and with unique know-how about the organization and logistical challenges present at each school, it was important to include them in this process to help create this new course. Furthermore, the students were able to ensure that their voice was represented; as a grassroots campaign that was started by student demand for such a course and program, the committee was able to ensure that the end product in place catered to the needs of its most important customer—the students themselves.

Creating Nuvention: Medical Innovation—The Steering Committee Builds a Start-Up

With all of the directors in place, the faculty and student combined steering committee began its first official meeting in December of 2006, with the daunting task of putting together the entire course and program under a tight timeline. In true start-up fashion, a Gantt chart was created by the engineering students, outlining all of

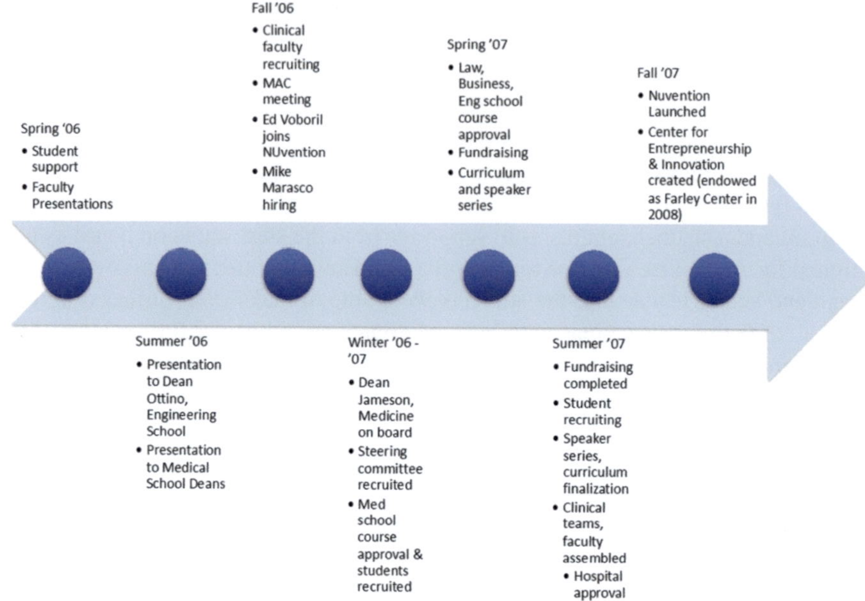

Fig. 10.6 NUvention development timeline from inception to launch, Spring '06 to Fall '07

Fig. 10.7 Initial LSIP/NUvention Steering Committee Organizational Structure 2007–2008

Organizational structure

- <u>NUvention Chairperson:</u> Ed Voboril, Chairman,
  - Greatbatch (NYSE-GB), Executive-in-Residence/Faculty and alumnus, McCormick School of Engineering and Applied Sciences
- <u>Clinical Faculty Director:</u> Patrick McCarthy
  - Chief of Cardiothoracic Surgery, NMH
- <u>Feinberg School of Medicine Co-Director(s):</u> Dean David Johnson
  - Assoc. Dean for Research Operations
- <u>Kellogg Graduate School of Business Director :</u> Alicia Loffler
  - Director of Kellogg Center for Biotechnology
- <u>Northwestern University Law School Director:</u> Clinton Francis
  - Professor of Law and Intellectual Property
- <u>McCormick School of Engineering Director:</u> Michael Marasco
  - Associate Professor and Director of McCormick Center for Entrepreneurship and Innovation
- <u>NUvention Founders / Student Directors:</u>
  - Swami Gnanashanmugam and Neel Patel – Feinberg/Medicine,
  - Todd Melby - Kellogg,
  - James Sulzer - McCormick,
  - Ash Nagdev – NU Law

the various elements that needed to be completed, the timelines for completion, and the work was divided amongst faculty and students alike (Fig. 10.8).

The curriculum and syllabus needed to be created, the speaker series needed to be recruited and arranged, course approval at each school needed to be secured, logistical issues such as gaining approval for students from all of the non-medical schools to gain hospital access for clinical immersion needed to be navigated, students from each school needed to be recruited and an application process formed, and last but certainly not least, funding for the course needed to be secured, all within 9 months.

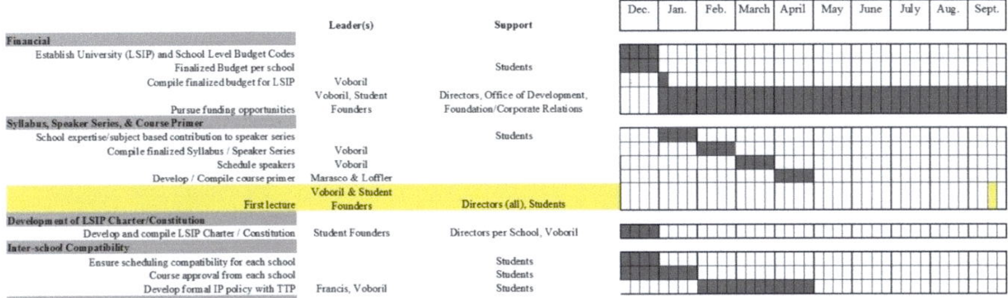

Fig. 10.8 Excerpt from LSIP/NUVention Gantt Chart, Early Winter 2007

As discussed previously, for the course to be successful, it had to be a self-sustaining entity, with a steady funding source that didn't draw from existing coffers within the university. The committee realized that to draw from existing funding sources inevitably meant competing with other pre-existing entities on campus that may have been dependent upon that funding, which would have meant opposition from the beginning to the establishment of the program. The committee thus focused on extramural grant funding opportunities, and industry funding. Initially, a NCIIA grant for a novel course was formulated by Professor Marasco and the students, however this bid for funding was ultimately unsuccessful. Realizing that grant funding timelines were too long, too cumbersome, and too onerous to fund such an educational program in such a short period of time, the committee quickly regrouped and focused on finding industry sponsorship for the program.

The plan was to secure 10, $25 K, unrestricted educational grants from a variety of different medical technology companies, with the ability to renew these grants from each company on a yearly basis, to continue to fund the program every year (Table 10.1). Each industry partner, in turn, would be invited to join the advisory board for the program, and would be invited to the mid-term and final presentations of the program.

The pitch to industry for funding relied on a few factors. One such factor was that there was a successful predicate in Stanford Biodesign, that some of the industry donors had already funded, that the committee was able to point to, and that modifying and replicating a similar program here at Northwestern would yield similar beneficial results. Additionally, one of the interesting differences between the program and Stanford Biodesign was that in each year, multiple clinical areas would be represented. Thus, a company like Stryker, with a predominantly orthopedic business, would be funding a program that, every year, would yield a team and a project focused on orthopedic innovation. In this manner, with 8–10 teams per year, the vast majority of medical technology companies could be canvased for funding as every year there would be a project relevant to their interests in their given clinical space. For these industry partners, the benefit of the grants was not only access to the course and the output of the course via their presence at the final presentations, but an opportunity to develop human capital, as the direct output of the course was approximately 80 students, all with a strong interest and a very well-versed skill set in the medical device industry.

Given that the various steering committee members had a background of working with industry, the plan was to use their extensive network to contact industry leaders

Table 10.1 Preliminary budget and financial projections for LSIP/NUvention

Financial Projections for Life Science Innovation Program # of teams 10

Committee Model

	Faculty	Duties	Nominal Quarterly Cost[a]	Fringe Benefits[b] (%)	Total annual cost	5-year program cost
Directors	Kellogg	Invite speakers, evaluate deliverables, course admissions	$5000	24	$12,400	
	McCormick		$0	0	$0	
	Feinberg		$5000	24	$12,400	
	Law School		$5000	24	$12,400	
	Course administrator	Help guide teams, ensure proper communication between teams and faculty, work with faculty to organize syllabus and speakers	$7000	24	$17,360	
			Cost/team			
	Prototyping[c]		$10,000		$100,000	
	Facilities[d,e]		51%		$27,826	
	Total annual cost:				**$182,386**	**$911,928**

[a]Based on quarterly Kellogg Prof. salary of $20,000

[b]Fringe benefits based on projected FY07-08 from http://www.northwestern.edu/orsp/fringe.html

[c]Prototyping half of Stanford "Bird-Seed" of $25,000 to $30,000/team

[d]Facilities cost based on projected FY07 from http://www.northwestern.edu/orsp/p_fa_defined.html

[e]Facilities cost based on percentage of faculty salaries, not prototyping costs

Fig. 10.9 Initial NUvention Advisory Board, 2007–2008

- Baxter
- Edwards LifeSciences
- Covidien
- Boston Scientific
- Medtronic
- Greatbatch
- Abbott
- Moog
- J&J
- Symark
- Morgan Stanley
- Enterprise VC

whom they had worked with, and pitch the idea of funding the course to those leaders. In this manner, the initial LSIP/NUvention advisory board was created, and funding for the course secured over the span of the ensuing months (Fig. 10.9).

With the fundraising plan in place, work began on forming the curriculum and syllabus for the course. Leveraging his relationship with Dr. Paul Yock, Gnanashanmugam was able to secure a meeting and displayed the plan for the fledgling NUvention program that was being created at Northwestern. Delighted by this creation, Dr. Yock welcomed the program as a needed addition to the Biodesign ecosystem, and offered to help with sharing Biodesign resources and to help support the program. The Biodesign course primer, the predecessor to the Biodesign textbook, and course materials from Gnanashanmugam's enrollment in the course served as inspiration for the new course and curriculum. The faculty directors leveraged this content when needed, and inspired by this content, also created their own. Furthermore, additional Northwestern faculty were brought in to help add content to the course, and the course soon had a who's who of Northwestern faculty superstars signed on to teach various aspects of the course. For instance, noted professor and marketing guru Timothy Calkins from Kellogg was signed on to give the marketing lecture for the course, and design leaders like professor Richard Lueptow signed on to help mentor students in the protoyping lab. Thus, Northwestern's full gamut of teaching and educational resources were leveraged to provide top-notch teaching for the course. For additional areas that required outside, industry expertise, experts were flown in as part of the speaker series to add additional content; in this manner, speaker like Susan Alpert, Sr. Vice President for regulatory affairs at Medtronic, and Anne-Marie Lynch, Exec. Vice President of payment and health care delivery policy for ADVAMED, were brought in for additional expertise on regulatory and reimbursement topics (Fig. 10.10). In this manner, a curriculum and syllabus was for the course was created and implemented.

With a course structure thus in place, a course approval process had to be initiated and completed at each school to ensure that students were able to enroll in the course and receive appropriate course credit. Each faculty director from each school, with help from the student directors, initiated this process of submitting the course description and materials for approval and gaining school curriculum committee approval in advance of the course. Once approval was granted the course was officially on the books at each school, faculty directors and students began advertising and marketing the course to students. An application for students was created for review by the faculty directors, and the course began enrolling students in the early spring of 2007, beginning with the medical school. Targeting rising fourth year medical students, who needed to have their schedules and clinical clerkships planned well in advance, initially proved challenging. However, leveraging personal connections with their classmates, targeting clinical faculty mentors to recruit their talented medical students, and bringing in prominent faculty and dean support to marketing pitches for the new and novel class, the committee was able to attract 15–20 qualified applicants to the course, exceeding the initial estimate of 10 students from the medical school. After the medical school, similar processes were put in place at the engineering, business, and law school, whose students soon followed suit. The course thus in its first year actually exceeded capacity, and 11 teams of 6–8 students were created, rather than turning qualified student applicants away.

Finally, logistical challenges were addressed. For instance, Northwestern Memorial hospital had never had a structure in place to formally allow and credential law, business, and engineering students to shadow physicians in the clinics, wards, and operating rooms. Existing structures for visiting observers were modified and adapted to this purpose, and students were able to gain access to the hospital, and also to lockers and given scrub codes and temporary ID badges. In this

NUvention: Fall Quarter Schedule, 2007-08

Module	Fundamentals / Ideation	Fundamentals II / Ideation	Fundamentals III / Ideation	Market Research	Conceptual Design/ Intel Prop	Opportunity Assessment	Opportunity Finalization	Intel Proof/ Prototyping (NO CLASS)	Intellectual Property	Clin. & Regul./ Design Present.	Business Plan Overview (NO CLASS)	Prototyping Workshops	Winter Break
Class Date	9/26/07	10/3/07	10/10/07	10/17/07	10/24/07	10/31/07	11/7/07	11/14/07	11/21/07	11/28/07	12/5/07	12/12/07	
Class Location	Lurie-Baldwin	Lurie-Hughes	Lurie-Hughes	McGaw-Daniel	Lurie-Hughes	Lurie-Baldwin	Lurie-Hughes	McGaw-Daniel	TBD	Lurie-Baldwin	McGaw-Daniel	TBD	
Faculty Lead	Al	Lueptow	ALL	Loffler/Schieffer	Lueptow/Francis	Volbert/Mansoor Loffler	Al	Francis/Lueptow	Francis	McCarthy/Lueptow	Volbert/Mansoor Loffler	Lueptow	
Curriculum	-Welcome-Volbert -Faculty Intros -Syllabus-Mansoor -Clinical-McCarthy	-Design Planning-Lueptow -IP/Patent Overview-Francis	-Regulatory and Reimbursement-McCarthy -Marketing-Calkins	-Customer Driven Prod. Dev -Customer Insight Tools -Market Potential	-Prod Dev Process -Customer-focused Innovation -Transferring Needs -Patent Searching-Francis	-Jonas vs. Business Opportunities -Opportunity Sizing	Elevator Pitch Presentations	-Patents vs. Trade Secrets -Patent Protection -Patent Infrng 022 -Fol Forty/Fol Offer	Patent Search Workshops	-FDA 101 -501(K) Process	Business Plan 101	Teams to meet with Design Committee prototype plan	
Faculty Teaching	Mansoor/Volbert/McCarthy	Lueptow/Francis	McCarthy/Calkins	Schieffer	Lueptow/Francis	Volbert/Mansoor Pier	Al Faculty Directors/Advisory Board invited	Francis Lueptow	Francis	McCarthy Lueptow	Loffler/Mansoor	Rich Lueptow Peter Campbell	
Guest Speaker	Bill Sanford Founder, STERIS		Amy Cunliffe, SVP Government Affairs ADVAMED		Craig Burroughs, IDEO	Michael Liang, Baird Venture Partners				-Susan Alpert Medtronic	Marc Galetti, Longitude Capital		
Deliverable				90 Clinical Needs	-Needs Prior Matrix -Product Concept & Goal -User Scenario	-Preliminary Pl. Pitch -Class Elevator Pitch	Elevator Pitch Presentations			Preliminary Design			
Project Team Efforts	Introductory Team meetings	-MD Shadowing -Needs Assessment	-MD Shadowing -Needs Assessment	-MD Shadowing -Needs Assessment	Elevator Pitch	Elevator Pitch	Elevator Pitch	Patent Searching Prototyping	Patent Searching Prototyping	Student Prototyping	Student Prototyping	Student Prototyping	Student Prototyping

NUvention: Winter Quarter Schedule, 2007-08

Module	Mid-Course Correction	Market Research Workshop	Clinical & Regulatory	Business Plan Marketing	Business Plan Strategy	Prototype Presentations	Business Plan Financing	Business Plan Legal	Business Plan Getting Started	Business Plan Dry Run	Investor Presentations
Class Date	1/9/08	1/16/08	1/23/08	1/30/08	2/6/08	2/13/08	2/20/08	2/27/08	3/5/08	3/12/08	3/19/08
Class Location	Jacobs 1246	Allen Center 342	Jacobs 1246	Jacobs 1246	Jacobs 1246	Jacobs 1246	Jacobs 1246	Jacobs 1246	Jacobs 1246	Jacobs 1246	Allen Center
Faculty Lead	Volbert/Mansoor	All	McCarthy/Volbert	Calkins	Loffler/Francis	ALL	Volbert/Mansoor	Francis	Volbert/Mansoor	All	All
Curriculum	-The Long Haul -Failure Learning -Overcoming Obstacles	NO CLASS Workshop from 12-6	-Code of Conduct -Conflict of Interest -Reimbursement -Early Adoption	-Creating Your Marketing Plan	-Business Model -Competitive Assessment -Exit Strategy -Value Chain Management		-Raising Money -Financing sources -Valuation -Term Sheets -Exit Strategy	-Patent Filing -Business/Invest Structure -Licensing -Managing Patent Infringement	-Bootstrapping vs Full On -Organization -Planning -Governance		
Faculty Teaching	Mansoor/Volbert	Z3 Associates	McCarthy/Volbert	Calkins	Loffler		Mansoor Volbert	Francis	Mansoor Volbert	All Faculty Directors	All Faculty Directors/Advisory Board
Guest Speaker	Bill Storts, Abroad		-Advamed -Anne Marie Lynch-Payment & Delivery -Chris White-General Counsel	No Guest	Andrew Cittadine CEO, American BioOptics		Sandy Thompson Morgan Stanley	No Guest	Entrepreneur /ISA		
Deliverable				Relevant Art Prior Analysis	Close to Final Prototypes		Intellectual Capital & Value Chain Mgt Plan	Patent Claims Draft		-Presentation Draft -Business Plan Doc Draft -Final Patent Claims & Spec -Prototype/Proof of Concept	-Final Presentation -Final Business Plan Doc -Final Patent Claims & Spec -Final Prototype/Proof of Concept
Project Team Efforts	Student Prototyping	Student Prototyping	Prototyping Business Plan	Prototyping Business Plan	Prototyping Business Plan		Business Plan	Business Plan	Business Plan	Business Plan	

Fig. 10.10 NUvention course schedule including faculty curriculum, guest speakers, and deliverables Fall and Winter 2007–2008

fashion, all manner of logistical issues were handled in a "just-in-time" method by the students and faculty directors, including coordinating parking for students who ordinarily did not travel between the two campuses, and adjusting course timings to accommodate the shuttle bus between campuses and the four different academic calendars of each school.

Finally, the unwieldy, preliminary name of the "Life Sciences Innovation Program" had to be modified in a manner becoming of Northwestern and the Kellogg's school of management's excellent reputation in marketing and advertising circles. A search for a new name was initiated, and the committee settled upon calling the new program NUvention, a nod to Northwestern University (NU), its new program, and the goal of inventing new technologies. And thus, via a whirlwind of productivity and herculean, group effort, the prototype NUvention: Medical Innovation course was created, just in time for the Fall quarter of 2007. The subtitle "Medical Innovation" was specified due to the intention of expanding NUvention to other fields, which at present has been accomplished very successfully, with over eight courses spanning multiple disciplines.

Section 2: *NUvention* Evolution and Present Day Structure

As mentioned earlier, The *NUvention*: Medical Innovation program is a two quarter, interdisciplinary course involving students from the Feinberg School of Medicine,

McCormick School of Engineering, Pritzker School of Law and Kellogg School of Management, that is currently in its 13th year. The students come together as a team with representation from each school, identify unmet health care needs, and with an entrepreneurial bent, develop solutions to address those needs, typically in the form of medical devices or, more recently, healthcare information technology solutions. During this process, each team develops a prototype, an investor presentation and a business plan. Where appropriate legal licensing and intellectual property filings are also made. The core principles of the course revolve around bringing together multidisciplinary teams, performing primary ethnography to identify unmet health care needs and business opportunities, and adopting an entrepreneurial approach to develop commercially viable solutions to address those unmet needs.

The classes are held once a week on Wednesday evenings. The fall quarter classes are held on the downtown Chicago campus at either the medical or law school and the winter quarter classes are held on the Evanston campus at either the engineering or business schools. The weekly classes span 3 h, and are typically divided into three parts: The first hour usually consists of a lecture/discussion from the faculty members covering the assigned readings and the topic for the week, followed by the second hour, which consists of a lecture/discussion session by an invited speaker who is an industry expert in the topic. These experts share their experiences and the lessons they have learned over their professional career in order to impart a "real world" perspective on the relevant topic. Followed by a short break, the last hour is allocated for the team time to allow the teams to meet and work on their class projects. Each team is assigned a faculty advisor who often participates in these meetings.

The Faculty Committee, composed of a faculty representative from each school, provides overall governance and guidance to the course. Examples of faculty committee responsibilities include curriculum development, financial oversight and addressing issues with regards to intellectual capital creation. The faculty representative from each school has primary responsibility for the students from their respective school and is ultimately responsible for assessing their students' performance and assigning grades. Each student is evaluated based on a combination of team assignments (approximately 2/3rd of the grade) which are project related and individual assignments plus participation (approximately 1/3rd).

The class started over a decade ago during the 2007–2008 with the teams focusing their projects within the broad specialty areas in modern medicine. These included Cardiovascular Surgery, Orthopedic Surgery, General/Minimally Invasive surgery, Urology, Neurosurgery, Radiology & Interventional Radiology, Ophthalmology, Emergency Medicine, Orthopedics and Otolaryngology. While initially the focus was on medical device development, over the course of the past decade, teams have increasingly shifted to include solutions in the healthcare services space with an emphasis on information technology. This shift is consistent with industry trends, given the increasing role health care information technology is playing in shaping the health care industry and the substantial increase in early stage capital investing in this area.

The Fall quarter primarily focuses on team formation as well as finding and screening numerous market opportunities for unmet needs. During this phase the classes target clinical and overall industry trends, customers and stakeholders, what private industry is thinking and where they are placing their bets, flows of early stage capital and design thinking and prototyping. These classes are driven by case studies and discussions and are designed to assist the teams in effectively narrowing down their prospective ideas.

During the ideation stage, clinical shadowing plays a pivotal role in giving the students a first-hand experience of how health care is delivered on the ground level and how their innovative ideas might be used to in improve health care. To prepare for this the students complete the paperwork required to shadow at the Northwestern Memorial Hospital and Lurie Children's Hospital, before the start of the class. Both are located adjacent to Northwestern's Chicago campus. Over the years, students have shadowed different areas in these hospitals spanning from ER rooms to surgical departments.

Over the past few years in addition to clinical subspecialty centered ethnography, students have also been exposed to the overall workings of the healthcare machine, gaining insights into overall hospital form and function, ambulatory care models, and the like. To facilitate this, during the Fall quarter, in addition to the typical immersion opportunities in the OR, wards, and clinics, shadowing sessions are organized for the students to meet the people working in Hospital logistics and innovation departments to discuss the problems they are facing that are in need of a newer, innovative approach. As a part of the class, the students are required to report on their observations and insights gained during their shadowing trips.

During this term, after identifying a range of unmet clinical needs and potential business opportunities, the students begin screening these needs in order to narrow them down to those they believe are the most commercially viable They are asked to compile their three most promising ideas with a description covering pertinent details such as medical need, market opportunity and their prospective deliverable product/service. These are subsequently presented as potential projects to external and internal guests which include the faculty members, medical device industry veterans, and the NUvention advisory board. The main purpose of the meeting is to provide feedback on the feasibility of the ideas including potential pitfalls, opportunities, etc., and to help the teams narrow their focus to one project for the remainder of the course. They are required to "pitch" this idea to the course advisors at the end of the term.

In the winter term, the classes are held in the Evanston campus. With a business idea selected, the students gear up for the next phase which addresses the challenges that the business will face and provides some guidance on how to implement their idea. The first step is market validation of the ideas by the teams. The teams are required to reach out to stakeholders, buyers, consumers etc. related to their idea in order to help understand the impact their idea will have on the market and who the key decision makers really are. The primary purpose of this market validation is for the teams to realize the how viable their idea is, and based on the feedback received from these varied parties, the teams get the opportunity to (and almost always do) modify their solution. Other challenges covered in the term (in addition to the prototype) include regulatory, reimbursement, business model issues, marketing and distribution, raising capital and business formation.

Each school's students contribute a domain-specific knowledge that enhances the overall project and the effectiveness of the team. The first part of the course typically leverages the medical school and clinical resources, such as immersion opportunities, to find significant market needs and resulting business opportunities. As the course progresses, domain expertise from the other schools becomes increasingly into focus, as the teams prepare for the final deliverables. A prime example is the prototype or the minimally viable product, an important component of the class, which is spearheaded by the engineering students on the team.

The McCormick School of Engineering has labs scheduled for its students, which are open to the non-engineering students as well. Topics cover basic shop training to ensure safety and teach the students to operate equipment such as lathes, mills, band saws and CNC machinery to develop their prototype. The product development process is carried out in an iterative manner and the labs are shaped accordingly. Topics such as 3D printing, laser cutting, CAD based software are covered, in addition to, more recently, topics such as software mockup-based development and electronics based development.

The Kellogg School of Management conducts dedicated supplementary classes in the winter quarter to assist students to work on developing the appropriate business model and the financials projections including costs required in the final deliverables. The final investor presentation and business plan need to make a convincing case that the idea is financially viable, fundamental to each team's chances of successfully landing future funding opportunities once the idea is out of the classroom into the dynamic startup-based ecosystem.

Additionally, The Legal Lab within the course for the Pritzker students addresses several issues that a start-up in the medical innovation domain needs to consider, including the following:

1. Entity formation: the different types of legal entities that a start-up should consider when deciding on its legal form: comparison of the different advantages, inconveniences, and costs
2. Patent searches: how to conduct an effective patent search, and issues to consider when you wish to patent your invention.
3. Trademarks and other IP: how to conduct Trademark and copyright searches, and protect project intellectual capital.
4. Investment: What are the legal ramifications surrounding different types and phases of investments a start-up company should expect and research regarding issues to consider for each type of investment.

This coursework is practical and allows a Law student to have a practical guideline of the issues to consider when assisting a start-up.

With the focus in the second half of the class shifting towards execution strategy for their ideas, the students work on a business plan and a final pitch for the class. This business plan serves as a final report and includes an executive summary, which serves as an important document designed to help locate potential investors. This plan thoroughly covers the market opportunity and the associated risks and challenges, covering important factors such as technical challenges, intellectual property, reimbursement strategy, and clinical and regulatory pathway. At the final presentation, the students present their ideas to an array of medical device industry experts with extensive experience. This process further leverages resources available at Northwestern and around the Chicago area in order to help the teams further develop the business ideas that they envisioned just a few months previously.

One such example of NUvention Medical's success is Briteseed, LLC, which was born during the 2011–2012 NUvention Medical class. Working in the domain of smart surgical tools, Briteseed has now successfully completed its seed round funding have raised \$2.7 M in equity financing and \$1.15 M in non-dilutive grants.[9]

A number of other companies originated in *NUvention: Medical Innovation*, in addition to medical device products that have been commercialized via licensing opportunities. In an interesting aside, the *NUvention: Medical Innovatio*n model of incorporating multidisciplinary teams, performing ethnography and needs finding, and developing entrepreneurial, innovative solutions with commercial potential to address those needs, has been translated into other courses outside of health care offered by the Farley Center for Entrepreneurship and Innovation at the McCormick school of Engineering. So far, nine other successful NUvention courses are offered: NUvention Arts, NUvention Web + Media, NUvention Energy, NUvention Transportation, NUvention Analytics, NUvention Therapeutics, NUvention Materials Science, NUvention Arts, and NUvention Wearables.

Section 3: Lessons Learned

The various chapters of this textbook have surely inspired the reader to pick up the mantle of innovation and pursue their own medical technology ideas to the benefit of patients. Perhaps they have even inspired a few readers to take on the daunting task of creating a program to teach and foster medical technology innovation within their section, department, academic medical center, or university. Even further, perhaps it has inspired a handful of readers to create and develop a multi-disciplinary, multi-institutional innovation and entrepreneurship program, similar to Northwestern's NUvention program. But, where does one begin? How does one go about creating a medical technology innovation program, within their respective institution?

The following section will dissect the experience of creating such a program in NUvention, and offer some critical lessons learned and insights into how and why NUvention was able to be created, in the hope that such a discussion will be useful to the reader interested in developing a similar program at their academic institution. It is the hope of the authors that these lessons and insights may have some applicability to the reader's own situation and surroundings, and while by no means are the following lessons meant to be a definitive treatise on how to start such a program, they do serve as insights in how a group of determined individuals succeeded in

---

[9] Briteseed Information sheet.pdf.

building one such program, and may offer at least one path or way in which one might go about achieving this daunting task.

In retrospect, a number of critical elements enabled the establishment of NUvention.

Fertile soil—one such element is that Northwestern already had talented schools of engineering, medicine, law, and business in place. In addition, in Chicago, a number of industry resources and outside resources were also in place. This presence of fertile soil, so to speak, was instrumental to the development of NUvention. Had elements been lacking, it likely would have been much more difficult to pull together all of the necessary components to build such a program.

Timing—A number of critical factors aided with the timing of the development of this program. Start-up culture and fostering innovation was a hot topic, undoubtedly buoyed by the success of universities like Stanford and start-ups like Hewlett-Packard, Yahoo, Google, and others that emerged from the university. Northwestern had just experienced a tremendous windfall in IP licensing from Lyrica, and this was an eye-opening event across the university, leading to more interest in trying to develop and commercialize intellectual property created across the University. The arrival of med-tech innovators in various schools across campus lead to a critical mass of like-minded, innovators and entrepreneurs who could support such a program; One such example was the formation of entities like the Bluhm Cardiovascular Institute and with it, leaders like Dr. Patrick McCarthy, whom had experience in successful licensing of medical device products. In this manner a critical mass of innovators had been achieved at the various schools; these innovators could thus then be connected to create such a program.

Student Leadership—a unique and critical element to the success of NUvention was that it arose from students. Whereas an administrator or faculty-driven model may have become a turf war between schools, a grassroots model driven by students, the customer base of the university, provided a neutral foundation. The students were willing to evangelize other students and faculty members to the cause, without conflicts of interest, fear of failure or loss of reputation. The curiosity, flexible schedule, energy, naiveté and audaciousness led to dozens of key meetings in just a few months. Fundamental to the solving of the collective action problem that was bringing together all of the constituents, the enthusiasm and energy to do such a potentially unrewarding, high risk, tedious task was a critical element that the students brought to the table.

If we can bring everyone together, will you join us?—this was the critical phrase at the end of every one of those pitches in the spring of 2006. Every member of the faculty told the students how impossible it would be to bring together all these resources, how much work it would be, etc. The students didn't fight that notion, but simply asked, if we managed to pull it off, would you join? In that way, students were able to get a commitment from faculty. Likely most faculty thought that they'd never see the students ever again, and that they would go nowhere fast. When the students eventually were successful, in a surprise turn of events, they were then compelled by the success to join, as promised.

Leadership—While student leaders like Gnanashanmugam and Sulzer were crucial to recruiting and aligning all of the stakeholders, the critical leadership of

Marasco is what made the course a reality. While the other faculty steering committee members had a number of full time responsibilities, Marasco was able to, in the position created for him by the Dean, devote a larger share of his time and energy to leading the team that formed NUvention. The gravitas leant to this by Voboril, who was chairman to Marasco's CEO, was another critical element to enable him, as a more junior faculty member, to lead a group of veteran faculty members to create this course. In turn, the leadership from the faculty steering committee—itself a group of talented individuals—who were willing to work together as a team to create something great together—and in this manner be led by students and faculty, was also instrumental to the creation of the course.

Key supporters—The program would not have been possible had it not been for the key supporters throughout this process. The faculty directors were instrumental to the development of the course, and the faculty members that didn't become directors, but never the less supported the course, with guest lectures and other content. Support from organizations like ITEC and IBIO were instrumental as well, as with that support, the core group could point to external organizations that validated the program they were trying to build. The support from Dean Ottino of Engineering, and the willingness to take a chance on a group of students, presenting to the advisory council meeting for the school, spoke volumes of the support. Following up this support with tangible action, by hiring two faculty members in Voboril and Marasco, was another critical step that showed to the other schools that the Engineering school meant business. That this support was in turn echoed by Dean Jameson of Medicine, added momentum to the movement and helped ensure that the remaining schools would also join in time.

Peer pressure—the involvement of the Engineering school compelled the medical school to join. That then compelled Kellogg, and in turn the law school. No one wanted to be left out without a dance partner. The same principle held true within the clinical realm. When one surgical department came on board, all the others wanted to join. When the surgeons came on board, the ER docs and radiologists and internal medicine physicians wanted in too. This fear of missing out, and the domino effect of seeing others join in, created an element of peer pressure that ensured that all the parties came together to join the program.

Luck—Often times, for programs like this to come to fruition, luck plays a hand. The McCormick advisory meeting and the enthusiastic reception from the group, mandating that the course be created and the timing of events of the unfortunate house fire in Voboril's house, and the opportunity that led to be able to recruit him to work on NUvention were some examples of some of the luck that made such a course happen.

Pointing to an existing successful predicate—the success of Stanford's Biodesign program, and the fact that this program would be borrowing from and modifying an already successful model, gave instant credibility to this initiative; without this success, it is likely that the concept would never have been able to succeed.

An Expanding Pie funding strategy—rather than competing for existing financial resources within the university (fixed pie), the course relied upon gaining funding from outside sources, thus expanding the overall funding pool for the university as a whole (expanded pie). This was critical to the success, as early on in the process, the group didn't have to ask for money from within the institution, rather, they could position the program as a way to grow the business so to speak, and to gain more funding from outside.

Designing a win-win situation—Inherent within the design of the program was the plan to create a symbiotic situation for all the stakeholders. Students not only received course credit, but were exposed to different parts of the university they otherwise would never experience, connect with people from the medical device world, and potentially launch a start-up. For faculty, the equal ownership model assured that they would get credit for creating and teaching such a unique course. For clinical faculty, their participation lead to the possibility of being involved in a novel medical innovation and the ensuing contribution to their field, the dream of any academic clinician. For leadership, paving the way for all these parties to participate was a small cost in lieu of the benefit the program provided in terms of enhancing the prestige and stature and IP portfolio of their school and the university. And for Industry, this was a small price to pay to develop talent, and potentially gain access and insight into novel technology at its infant stages. That the costs of participating were far outweighed by the benefits for all the stakeholders involved, was crucial to the program's success.

Avoiding fool's gold—often, a suggestion would be made to take a smaller step such as to create a pilot program, consisting of just a few students and one clinical team, for instance. This temptation was avoided at all costs. A pilot program would lack all the resources of the full program, and would be inherently set up to fail in this regard. The goal was always to create an entire program, or none at all, and in this regard, the line was held.

Equal ownership—the fact that each school would be an equal partner was critical in the early stages. This ensured enthusiasm from all parties to give freely of resources, and ensured there was no jealousy amongst any one group over the other, avoiding any favoritism or infighting.

Motivation—the group was able to tap into the motivation of the leadership to raise the prominence of their schools, to be ranked amongst the best institutions worldwide within their respective disciplines. Furthermore, industry leaders resonated with the plan that programs like this could help change the notion that the Midwest was an "innovation flyover zone" between the two innovative hubs in Silicon valley and Boston on the west and east coasts.

Teamwork—the program succeeded because no one person had to pull it all together. Each person brought their own unique talents to the table, and the program allowed them to build upon that to create something greater than the sum of its parts.

These were some of the critical factors that enabled a stalwart group of students to inspire physicians, academic faculty, and institutional leadership, to create a lasting, multi-disciplinary, multi-institutional innovation and entrepreneurship program within an academic setting. It is the sincere hope of the authors, that this chapter and knowledge and insights that it provides will inspire, and perhaps help instruct, the reader to pick up the torch of innovation and to forge ahead and blaze new trails.

Chapter 11
Challenges to Academic-Industry Partnerships

Randy J. Seeley, Gregory N. Witbeck, and Michael W. Mulholland

Introduction

Never before has it been more important for those in academic medicine to interact with for-profit, industrial partners to address important unmet medical needs. Many of the challenges facing medicine require complex solutions that necessitate a combination of disciplines and technologies. Meeting this need requires diverse teams that can assess technical, medical, and market challenges to specific solutions. Additionally, it is clear that many large companies currently outsource much of their research and development work to outside entities including academic institutions. Academic investigators face increasing pressures to show their work has impact on patients and to provide stable funding to support diverse teams of researchers.

Academic research labs develop deep skill and knowledge bases that are often not fully utilized. Working with industrial partners can provide both diversity to the revenue stream of a lab and a path to bring the work to bear on human disease. However, such relations come with a number of important challenges that range from cultural to budgetary. Appropriate institutional support is necessary to realize the potential of these partnerships. We will review some of these challenges and what we have done in the Department of Surgery at the University of Michigan to help investigators find and successfully execute novel academic industrial partnerships.

As we will discuss further, many academic researchers view these relationships in a decidedly one-sided manner that sounds something like this. "My laboratory has generated hard-won ideas and now it is time to find someone to help us commercialize these into next generation therapies." This pathway is an important source of

R. J. Seeley (✉) · G. N. Witbeck · M. W. Mulholland
Department of Surgery, University of Michigan, Ann Arbor, MI, USA
e-mail: seeleyrj@med.umich.edu; germaine@med.umich.edu; micham@med.umich.edu

© Springer Nature Switzerland AG 2019
M. S. Cohen, L. Kao (eds.), *Success in Academic Surgery: Innovation and Entrepreneurship*, Success in Academic Surgery,
https://doi.org/10.1007/978-3-030-18613-5_11

innovation and potential revenue for academic researchers. However, this common scenario ignores the clear reciprocal needs of industrial partners to solve problems that are generated as they pursue their own ideas about potential new products. In many cases, industrial R&D uses contract research organizations (CRO) to fill gaps in research capabilities. The use of such CROs is likely to continue to grow.

Academic researchers can potentially play an important role in filling in the research gaps for industrial partners in work that might be termed "fee-for-service". This is especially important in highly specialized areas of research where building a research capability de novo for contract research simply doesn't make sense. Large sums of money are invested every year into building cutting-edge research capabilities at academic institutions. Those capabilities can be leveraged to provide important data back to industrial partners that facilitate their research efforts without the time and expense of building capabilities in the form of specialized equipment and training of personnel. This is particularly true when such capabilities are only needed on a limited basis rather than being a core part of an industrial R&D capability. Additionally, academic institutions are able to combine multiple types of these sophisticated capabilities into a single solution for an industrial partner. No CRO has the diverse sets of capabilities found at a large research university. The important point is that despite the availability of CROs, academic medical centers can benefit both their mission and their bottom lines by helping industrial partners solve specific R&D problems even when the academic center has not generated the technology or intellectual property being advanced.

Challenges to "Fee-for-Service" Work in Academic Medical Centers While the need for these types of academic-industrial relationships is clear, they face a number of important challenges in academic research institutions. These challenges extend from the level of the individual investigators to the multi-tiered bureaucracy that supports research and to the highest levels of leadership at academic institutions.

Culture

In American academic medical centers, relationships with industry have revolved around two broad areas of interest. The first form of interaction, expressed via traditional research grants or contracts, involves ideas generated by academic faculty with monetary support for ongoing development sought from an industrial sponsor. In this model, well-established concepts around intellectual property and publication practices apply. The second form of relationship is typified by the commercialization of novel ideas generated by academic faculty members. In most instances, the novel concept or product derives from the research work performed by faculty, with the idea, product, or device transferred for monetary compensation to an outside industrial entity for fuller development, testing, and eventual commercialization. These relationships are highly regulated, expressed via time-honored legal instruments, and are bureaucratic. The academic medical culture, evolved over many decades to accommodate these interactions, has become risk-averse, conservative, and restrictive. In short, full creativity is greatly inhibited.

Culture may be considered as "how we do things around here". While most organizations have a recognizable culture, its development is often an organic process that is at the same time unintentional and powerful. Given the importance of culture to the mission of academic centers, those that decide to make "innovation" a core value must evolve an innovative culture. Core values must be made explicit so that they may be expressed consistently.

A core tenet of an innovative culture is that the best work is done collaboratively at the intersection of different disciplines. Innovators deliberately seek research and innovation collaborators from other fields for each project. Continuous feedback and constructive criticism are also essential to culture change. Feedback must be shared with individuals and teams because impactful innovation is a team sport.

One vehicle for culture change employed at the University of Michigan is entitled the "Michigan Surgical Innovation Prize". The first installment of the $500,000 Prize program including novel curriculum and resources, and engaged over 40 surgeons, scientists, engineers, surgical residents, and medical students. These innovators focused their energies on development of ideas and surgical technologies that have potential to impact the care of surgical patients. The participants enrolled into a year-long program that guided them on how to navigate their ideas through the university and into the market.

In existence for the past 3 years, the Michigan Innovation Prize has developed programs and resources for faculty in Innovation and Entrepreneurship across the medical campus and the Department of Surgery has created one of the more advanced and tailored programs in existence. This success has stimulated change in other departments on the medical campus, leading other departments and centers to engage in their own innovation efforts. Together this effort has created a broad impact on the culture that brings into focus a wide array of commercialization activities.

The Accelerated Business Engagement program is a second example of culture change. There is an old adage that says: No margin, no mission. Just so: No margin, no culture change. This new approach to industry-academic collaborations is structured to provide a diversified revenue stream for supporting academic research. In every academic department, large investments have been made in the intellectual and physical infrastructure for research. The Accelerated Business Engagement model provides for a way to leverage those existing investments. We believe that this approach is complimentary to the more traditional models that commercialize discoveries from academic laboratories. Importantly, the Accelerated Business Engagement program facilitates industrial relationships that fit into the "fee-for-service" model. More detail about these activities will be described below. However, by setting up this organization, it sends an important message to individual investigators that this kind of work is valued and supported.

Finding Partners

A key challenge to providing services to industrial partners is to find entities that could utilize these services and make them aware of the potential capabilities. All CROs employ marketing/sales organizations that actively seek potential business in a variety of ways. While some individual academic investigators may have strong ties to potential industrial customers, many do not. How do we help investigators with important capabilities find industrial research partners who are willing to pay to gain access to these capabilities?

One key to successful implementation of the Accelerated Business Engagement initiative was the hiring of a Senior Director for Business Development. This individual was charged with identifying non-traditional revenue sources to support research activities in the Department of Surgery. The Senior Director for Business Development was to identify non-academic conferences that convened significant numbers of prospective industry and philanthropic professional foundation collaborators.

Conferences such as the Alliance for Regenerative Medicine's "Meeting on the Mesa" do not draw academic presenters but do serve as a focal point for many companies operating in the regenerative life sciences. These sorts of conferences provide opportunities for outreach. Such conferences routinely employ partnering software that allow attendees to identify organizations of interest and invite them to schedule 30 min meetings. The purpose of the meetings is to lay out assets and expertise on the part of the University and to review a wish-list of a company's specific interests in licensing opportunities as well as in learning about opportunities in academic research related to drug discovery, medical device development, diagnostics, etc. In FY 18, the first full year of the program, 54 such face to face meetings were scheduled by the Senior Director for Business Development, which resulted in ten follow-up campus visits and multiple PI meetings with University of Michigan faculty. Further discussions led to formalization of four material transfer agreements, three non-disclosure agreements, six patent filings, and three NIH SBIR grant applications. In the first quarter of FY 19, 65 face to face meetings have been conducted at three conferences, leading to many promising opportunities for upcoming campus visits, contract and sponsored research collaborations, grants, and other forms of partnership. The important point is that with a relatively modest investment, UM was able to rapidly start connections that can lead to commercialization and research activities including fee-for-service contracts.

Budgetary Challenges

Traditional research grants build a budget based almost entirely on the anticipated costs of the research. Most investigators have built an NIH-style budget where they estimate the amount of effort for personnel, costs of reagents, and services needed to accomplish the proposed research. Often these budgets can have time scales over multiple years that allow for stable funding of lab personnel. Budgeting for fee-for-service work is considerably different. By its nature, this type of work is more transient and will have ebbs and flows in the amount of work needed at any given time. This requires a very different approach to budgeting that is unfamiliar to most academic investigators. Rather than estimating the cost of the experiments, the clear focus must be on the value of the data that will be realized from those experiments. Important variables must be included in the calculation of value:

1. True costs. NIH budgeting only examines the incremental costs of doing specific experiments. It does not take into account the years of work that may have been required to build the appropriate experimental models and or techniques. Budgeting for fee-for-service agreements needs to include the costs to build and validate experimental models and approaches. It is often the case that millions of dollars in equipment, facilities and skilled labor go into developing an experimental model that an industrial partner may wish to access. Relatedly, what would be the cost of independently building this capability? How much time would it take? From the industrial partner's point of view these are key issues. The ability to access such a capability quickly and easily without the need for hiring personnel with highly specialized skill sets has enormous value. The cost charged to the industrial partner needs to reflect that value.

2. Increased value of a product or service. Will these data make existing intellectual property, product or service more valuable for the industrial partner? This can happen in a number of ways. Will these data speed a regulatory review? Time is money and speeding up needed approvals for a product brings value. Will this open up a product to new markets or indications? If so, what is the size of that market? Will these data provide a useful comparison to competing products? Insights that can be used in the further marketing of the product can help realize significant gains in market share. Finally, can this information be used to convince payers to cover the product or service? In a complicated health care system, such information can greatly increase sales/revenue for a product. Needless to say, the value of such outcomes need to be balanced by the likelihood of the outcome helping realize such value. Often experiments are being done precisely because something is unknown and both the technical and hypothesis-based risks must be used to discount the potential value.

3. Margin. Almost all fee-for-service work will involve at least some "opportunity costs". That is to say, personnel and other elements of a lab's capacity will need to be dedicated to executing these experiments. By definition that means that those individuals will not be doing experiments that are driving the scientific agenda of that laboratory. The price charged to the industrial partner needs to reflect these opportunity costs. Simply put, one needs to charge an amount that makes it worthwhile for the associated activities to accomplish the fee-for-service work. Such a margin should provide for enhanced abilities of a research lab to pursue its own research agenda.

4. Competition. Are there other labs/universities that can provide the same solutions? Will they do so at a lower cost? Needless to say, the more "generic" the service the more difficult it is to charge a premium. This is particularly the case when such services are provided by traditional CROs.

The bottom line is that a careful consideration of value needs to accompany the pricing of such fee-for-service work. It is often the case that academic investigators greatly under value their services. The result of this is that they charge too little and do not adequately derive the additional resources that would make these activities valuable to their own research agenda. This results in abandoning these activities before the benefits can be realized.

Another important aspect of budgeting is to be sure that adequate resources are dedicated to the marketing activities that bring in potential partners. From the initial planning stages of the Accelerated Business Engagement initiative, it was clear that a substantial travel budget would be necessary to adequately support the Senior Director for Business Development in reaching a series of conferences which matched the criteria of being primarily non-academic venues which drew large numbers of companies operating in the biomedical, device, and pharmaceutical space. It also, correctly, anticipated that additional conferences would come to the Senior Director's attention over the course of travel, so operation funds were set aside for airfare, lodging, and registration for five to six conferences annually, with additional support available to travel in pursuit of arising opportunities with new prospective philanthropic foundation partners outside the context of conferences. Institutional support needs to be provided for these activities to make individual investigators successful.

Procedural Challenges

The Accelerated Business Engagement program challenges many traditional practices of academic medicine. The willingness to forego intellectual property claims, proprietary handling of investigative data, potential lack of publication rights, and non-involvement of trainees are all contrary to traditional academic business practices. For such a program to be successful, unequivocal institutional support is crucial.

The most essential question: Is the activity research or a contract service? For the Accelerated Business Engagement program this issue is resolved using the decision tree presented below.

The following questions are used to outline and describe a proposed Contract Service arrangement. Contract Service Definition:

The provision of a good, service, or otherwise developed concept – involving repetitive, quantitative, non-experimental measurement under physically controlled conditions for which the data produced are expected to be within a predetermined range of value or of reproducibility – that may have benefit to the recipient.

The results generated in the performance of a contracted service(s) are required to be provided to the customer, will remain the sole and exclusive property of the customer, and may not be published by the University or University-employed researchers performing said service(s).

Who is the principal investigator of the proposed contract service? Who is the customer (data recipient) of the proposed contract service?

Questions: Yes or No
1. Is any intellectual property being generated by an employed researcher as a result of the proposed contract service? Intellectual property includes inventions, patents, trademarks, computer software, and copyrighted works.
If "NO", continue to question 2
2. Will trainees (including graduate and postdoctoral students) be used to facilitate the proposed contract service?
If "NO", continue to question 3
3. Is there any intention for the principal investigator to publish the results of the proposed contract service?
If "NO", continue to question 4
4. Does the proposed contract service utilize a previously established model or methodology (e.g. previously published study, considered general knowledge)?
If "YES", continue to question 5
5. Is the industry sponsor responsible for developing the experimental protocol(s) of the proposed contract service?
If "YES", continue to question 6

If the answers to the questions in Sect. II are any combination other than "NO" (question 1), "NO" (question 2), "NO" (question 3), "YES" (question 4), and "YES" (question 5) the proposed project does not qualify as an applicable contract service.

6. What is the overarching goal of the proposed contract service?

7. More specifically, what is being tested? That is, what is the expected outcome or objective for the proposed contract service?

8. Briefly describe the scope of the proposed contract service and timeline of expected results.

9. What deliverables are required, and to what degree will the results of proposed contract service be analyzed by the principal investigator? What technique(s) will be employed to model or display the results?

These questions constitute a set of guidelines that can aid in deciding whether this research activity belongs in this adapted model for academic-industry partnerships. This process has evolved into a standardized, re-usable, template form to which an agreed-upon Standard of Work can be appended. This significantly boosts efficiency in negotiating and formalizing contract research agreements because it obviates the need for each agreement to be painstakingly "hand-crafted" as a one-off type arrangement. A last consideration is to evaluate for industry contracts if a more favorable indirect rate could be negotiated with the University compared to the contracted rate used for federal research grants (which at many universities is upwards of 50–90% of direct cost value). The better this rate can be modified for industry contracts, the more value is added to an industry partner to engage in such an opportunity with an academic lab or institution.

Conclusion

Academic-industrial partnerships continue to evolve and our institutional approaches need to evolve as well. In particular, the great need to leverage the enormous capabilities housed in academic research centers to solve medical problems means that we need to think beyond the intellectual property out-licensing approach that has been the dominant approach for decades. The ability to provide "fee-for-service" capabilities for industrial partners provides a unique opportunity. While such relationships have significant challenges, they can provide an important source of revenues for individual laboratories and institutions that has not been fully realized. Such revenues can diversify and stabilize research money and allow for greater investment in the next generation of capabilities for academic research institutions.

Chapter 12
Funding Engineering/Surgical Partnerships to Accelerate Commercialization of Academic Medical and Surgical Innovations: The Coulter Model for Translational Partnership between Medicine, Engineering, and Industry

Thomas Marten

Introduction

According to Wikipedia, translational research is often used interchangeably with translational medicine and "bench to bedside" with the goal of de-risking and building off basic research to create new therapies, medical devices, and diagnostics [10]. This chapter will focus on leveraging academic translational research funding and funding program support to accelerate commercialization of innovative medical technologies invented at universities and academic medical centers by clinicians and engineers. The emphasis of discussion here will be on medical devices and clinical diagnostics.

As universities and academic medical centers are not typically structured, staffed, or financed to bring medical technologies through the product development and FDA approval process, a hand-off to a commercial entity at some point during research is required, in most cases, to enable commercialization and product launch. As such, in order to reach the "bedside" goal of translational research to bring new medical innovations into patient care as FDA approved products, incentives must be aligned for a commercial partner to invest in the technology and bring the innovation to market as a new medical device or diagnostic.

Ironically, academic translational research alone rarely reaches the "bedside" stage. Translational research programs typically focus on technical de-risking and demonstration of in-vitro or in-vivo animal proof of concept studies with benchtop or very

T. Marten (✉)
Coulter Translational Research Partnership Program, Department of Biomedical Engineering,
University of Michigan, Ann Arbor, MI, USA
e-mail: tmarten@umich.edu

© Springer Nature Switzerland AG 2019

M. S. Cohen, L. Kao (eds.), *Success in Academic Surgery: Innovation and Entrepreneurship*, Success in Academic Surgery,
https://doi.org/10.1007/978-3-030-18613-5_12

early stage prototypes. However, with the need to "exit" or "hand-off" technologies to a commercial entity in the form of a license of the intellectual property (IP) to an established medical device company (strategic) or to a start-up company who go on to raise venture capital (VC) or angel(A) investor financing to complete development, a solid business case, human proof of concept and/or more advanced product development is typically required to justify investing in academic medical and surgical innovations. Alternatively, experienced medical device entrepreneurs need to be identified who have an interest in working with the technology at an early stage, and capability of forming a new company and raising capital through economic development and other non-dilutive sources before reaching the venture "investibility" stage where adequate financing can be secured to continue development.

This chapter will propose an alternative approach to translational research, as exemplified by the UM-CP, that involves a transition from academic research to a new product planning and development project management approach, with early and often interactions with strategics and VCs to accelerate exits and earlier commercialization of academic medical and surgical innovations.

Challenges with Commercializing Medical and Surgical Innovations

Meeting Investor Needs

Achieving a medical innovation licensing exit from an academic center to a strategic or to a startup that raises VC/A financing is a monumental challenge for academic project teams, that is often underestimated by clinical and engineering faculty involved with innovation research. Medical device investing by strategics and VCs requires significant financing and assumption of high risk, with oftentimes lower returns than comparable investments in therapeutics or other healthcare innovations. Successful academic project licensing to VC-backed startups or strategics requires an understanding of the investor point of view in order to develop translational research strategies to enhance the probability of reaching an exit deal.

Strategics and VCs are keenly aware of the costs involved in developing FDA regulated medical devices, and the funding requirements they face before reaching their goals: FDA approval and revenues or sale of portfolio company developing devices. Medical device development costs vary widely, and little is published on actual development costs in the US. Data from a 2010 survey of 204 public and venture-backed medtech companies evaluated the costs to medtech companies of developing medical devices [4] (Fig. 12.1). While these findings may be outdated for 2019, they provide a clear demonstration of the magnitude of funding required to bring medical devices to market and have likely gone up since 2010.

The average cost to bring a 510 (k) FDA regulatory pathway device[1] to market was $31 M. As survey respondents made reference to requiring an Investigational Device Exemption (IDE) for 510(k) pathway devices, this indicates a survey

---

[1]For an overview of the FDA medical device approval process and pathways, visit https://www.fda.gov/ForPatients/Approvals/Devices/default.htm.

	510(k) ($M)	PMA ($M)
Concept to Clinical-ready protype	$7	$19
IDE to Clearance or Approval	$24	$75
Total	$31	$94

Fig. 12.1 Source: Makower et al. [4]

response bias towards companies developing novel and innovative devices that require clinical performance data, as opposed to simple 510(k) devices that are line extensions or minor improvements on existing devices that only require demonstration of substantial equivalence to an existing marketed medical device to obtain clearance for marketing without clinical data requirements. Hence the survey respondents were more likely to be representative of university spin-out startup companies developing innovative and novel medical technologies invented at academic medical settings.

One can argue that a startup that reaches the IDE stage may be "venture ready" for receiving venture capital financing. However, this still would require an average of $7 M to reach this stage, which exceeds typical funding raised through non-dilutive funding sources - National Institute of Health (NIH)- R01 or other federal grants, Small Business Innovation Research (SBIR) grants, Small Business Technology Transfer (STTR) grants or other non-dilutive economic development funding for startups.

For higher risk, Pre-Market Authorization (PMA) FDA pathway devices, the costs to reach the clinical-ready device stage are even higher at an average of $19 M, with a total $94 M required to reach FDA approval. Most early stage companies developing PMA devices require multiple rounds of VC financing, which present even higher risks for investors. These risks also pertain to strategics who would need to invest in the $100 M range to develop high risk devices that may fail in clinical trials or never gain the market acceptance required to realize an adequate return on investment.

Based on Silicon Valley Bank research [7] (Fig. 12.2) evaluating VC backed merger and acquisition (M&A) exits (VC backed company sales to strategics or initial public offerings), the majority of VC backed device companies developing 510(k) devices did not achieve exits until after FDA clearance for marketing. Hence, VCs had to hold on to these companies for a median time of over 9 years, and achieved a relatively low deal multiple or return on investment of only 3.6 times money invested. This is in clear contrast to PMAs and De Novo 510(k)s that generated nearly 7× returns with a median time to exit of only 5.5 years. However, biopharma M&As for therapeutics companies achieved over 12× returns from even lower investments and quicker times to exits on average.

The key points to consider: 510ks are least expensive and quickest path from bench to bedside, but for investors create a long road to an exit, with relatively low returns. PMA/De Novo 510(k)s present greater risks, but higher returns than 510(k)

2015 – 1H 2018	Number of Exits	Pre-FDA and CE Mark Approval Exits	Median Invested ($M)	Median Total Deal Multiple	Median Time to Exit (Years)
510(k) M&As	29	2 (7%)	$46	3.6x	9.1
PMA/ De Novo 510(k) M&As	22	20 (91%)	$45	6.8x	5.5
Biopharma M&As	60	60 (100%)	$37	12.5x	4.2

Fig. 12.2 VC Backed Device M&A By Pathway. Source: Silicon Valley Bank, Trends in Healthcare Investments and Exits Mid-Year 2018

s. However, biopharma M&As with similar risks lead to even higher returns with comparable investments and time horizons. Hence, VCs in general have a greater focus on therapeutics investing in the healthcare space. As such, one can see the challenges with attempting to raise VC financing for medical devices. However, a number of venture capital firms have expertise in investing in medical devices, and continue to invest in this space.

Strategics in the medical device space continuously look to enhance their product pipelines and portfolios, although more typically through acquisitions of entire companies compared to early stage licensing deals. These investors are unlikely to invest in device projects within academia or early stage companies with devices unless these devices are at the advanced development stage or at the FDA submission stage of development. By taking a new product planning and development approach while in academia, clinician and engineering teams can approach and occasionally reach this stage, but only with advanced knowledge of investor criteria for licensing and sharply focused efforts to meet these criteria. Each investor will have a unique set of criteria they need to see before investing. By understanding investor perspectives and criteria that investors (strategics or VCs) require prior to investing, academic medical researchers will be in a much better position to utilize translational research funding and support to achieve licensing exit goals.

Crossing the Valley of Death

When it comes to translational research and commercializing academic medical research and innovations, much has been written about the valley of death. Pienta refers to the valley of death in a 2010 review of the Michigan Coulter Translational Research Partnership program [5] and describes it as the funding and support gap between discovery stage and the point where strategics and VCs feel comfortable investing. The discovery stage is typically the early concept medical innovation

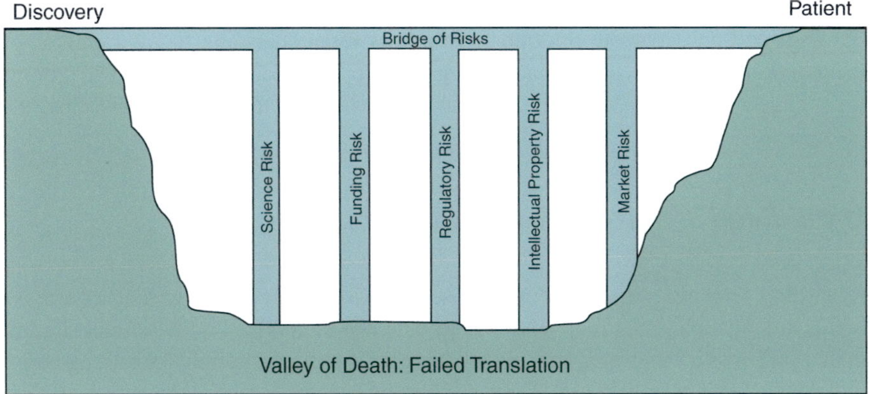

Fig. 12.3 Source: University of Michigan Coulter Program [5]

stage with bench top prototype proof of concept. This gap is where translational research funding has garnered significant attention and funding over the recent past.

Pienta refers to four main pillars of risk when traversing the valley of death: scientific, intellectual property (IP), market and regulatory. (Fig. 12.3) These four risks can be distilled into basic questions that guide investment decisions.

- *Scientific* or technical risk addresses the question, "Will the device work as intended?" This includes demonstrating both pre-clinical proof of concept through bench studies and animal models, along with human proof of concept through clinical studies to demonstrate both efficacy and safety.
- *IP* addesses the question, "Can we own this?" Is the concept patentable with claims that create an effective blocking strategy preventing future competitors from developing similar devices? Will we have freedom to operate and not infringe on other issued patents once the final product is developed and marketed? IP is often an early "deal breaker" with investors if a concept is considered non-patentable, or is in a crowded space with many issued or expired patents.
- *Market* addresses the question, "What is the intended use and indication for use? Is the unmet medical need for this indication great enough to convince health care providers/insurers to use/pay for new product? and "Is the target market big enough and sustainable enough to justify investment?"
- *Regulatory* addresses the question, "What is the pathway the FDA will use to regulate the device?" With the most common question, "Can this be '510(k) able'?" In other words, can the device be developed at a reasonable cost?

Translational research has been historically focused on risk reduction. However, complete de-risking is not feasible in an academic setting. In fact, complete de-risking may not be feasible in a large company setting with much larger budgets, and may not occur until after the product is on the market. Thus, risk mitigation is more of a continuum where it's better to think of screening at the translational research stage, with an eye towards periodic reevaluation of risks throughout the development process.

Answering the "smell test" early with an appropriate level of due diligence to identify red flags and unacceptable risks up front allows researchers and funding entities to make funding decisions and focus funding and support on addressing specific criteria (due diligence requirements) that target investors will need to see before investing.

If you Build it, Make Sure they Come!

Regarding screening, it's common to observe an insular approach to market assessments amongst clinician innovators. Who better to understand unmet medical need than a surgeon or other medical specialist facing a particular clinical challenge on a daily basis? This may lead to a "Field of Dreams" perception with the notion "If you build it, they will come." While this makes for a great movie plot, it is ill-advised when developing new medical products. In the movie *Field of Dreams*, a voice tells the main character to build a baseball field in the middle of his cornfield in Iowa, despite the risk of going into financial ruin and losing the farm. Without fully understanding the implications, he plows under a large portion of his corn field and builds a baseball field. This is highly analogous to academic medical innovators who devote significant time and resources on conducting research related to a product concept, or leaving academia or residency programs to start companies to commercialize technologies without fully understanding whether investors will "come" or in this case invest or license technology.

Different healthcare systems and health care settings have different needs, and healthcare providers in these settings will have varying perceptions of potential new solutions. Reimbursement and budgets to pay for new products vary greatly as well. Conducting market research with external audiences and socializing concepts with investors and strategics is crucially important to ensure any new product solution emanating out of medical innovation work meets the needs of target investors and customers.

License vs. Startup?

Academic medical inventors seeking to commercialize IP based technologies out of universities are faced with two options: (1) form a new company to commercialize the medical technology or (2) license the IP to an existing company that will then bring the product concept to market. Forming a company has many advantages (beyond the scope of this article) and often allows the inventors to remain involved with product development in an advisory, if not managerial capacity. However, this most often requires building a team and raising capital from VC or angel investors. Strategics on the other hand prefer to license or acquire product concepts close to the FDA approval stage or on the market and generating revenue. The exception occurs when the concept fills a strategic void or is highly complementary to corporate strategic direction. Licensing university based medical device concepts to strategics is analogous to "threading a needle" to meet their strategic needs and licensing requirements, and requires a high level of interactions with potential strategic suitors long before a licensing event occurs.

If academic medical innovators meet these conditions while the research is still pre-license at the university, licensing to a strategic can occur before a company is formed. In this case, the medical device company will take over development after licensing and be well positioned with resources, know-how, and infrastructure to bring the licensed product concept through the FDA and into the market. Licensing agreements between universities and strategics are structured to incentivize companies to bring licensed technologies to market within an acceptable time frame, and avoid scenarios where companies under-resource or abandon development.

"The Team, The Team, The Team!": Bo Schembechler, former Michigan football coach

If academic medical innovators elect to form a new company around a university-based technology, execution adds a significant new layer of risk. New companies formed around a technology typically have no existing infrastructure or management team. In such cases, this all then needs to be built or outsourced. Management execution to accomplish fund raising and product development is equal in importance to the technology itself. VCs only invest in companies, and as the old saying goes, they bet on the "jockey as well as the horse". A recent survey of 885 VCs found that with healthcare investing, "The Team" was the most important factor that contributed to successful investments, and equally important to the technology as the top factor contributing to failed investments (Fig. 12.4). As such, finding the right CEO is arguably the most important decision academic medical innovators face when striving to go the VC backed startup exit route [3].

Key takeaways – Predetermining the most likely exit path and identifying interested investors before or in the early stages of seeking funding will greatly increase odds of achieving an exit. While the four pillars of risk generally apply, investing criteria are specific to each type of investor. As such, mapping out an exit strategy before seeking translational research funding can help with risk prioritization and with setting funding milestone goals that address investor top concerns.

The Coulter Model Partnership Program and the University of Michigan Coulter Translational Research Program

The University of Michigan Coulter Translational Research Partnership Program (UM-CP) is a translational research funding program at the University of Michigan that funds UM faculty translational research projects. The program is funded by the proceeds of a $20 million endowment from the Wallace H. Coulter Foundation (WHCF), with a match from the UM Medical School and UM College of Engineering. The program is housed within the UM Biomedical Engineering (BME) Department.

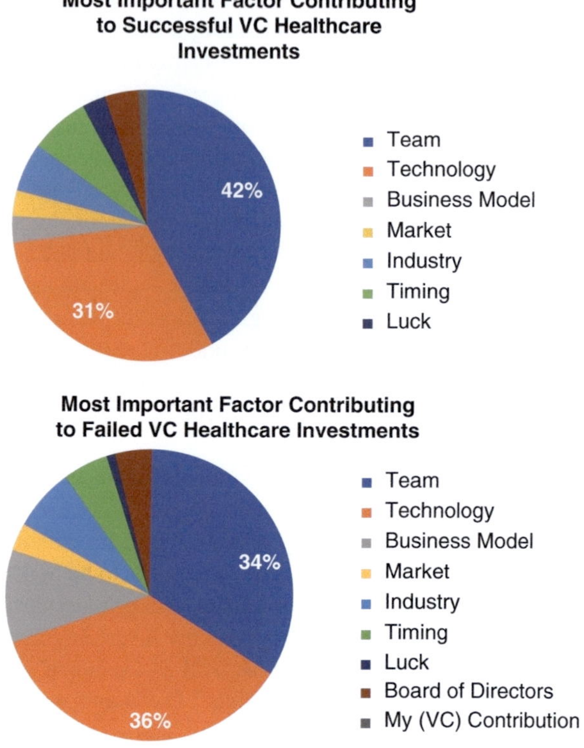

Fig. 12.4 Source: Gompers, et al., How Do Venture Capitalists Make Decisions?, NBER Working Paper No. 22587, Sept 2016

The goal of the program is to bring medical innovations into healthcare through a commercial entity. These goals are codified into 5-year rolling metrics that include a pre-specified number of projects that culminate with direct licensing of IP to strategics and/or licensing of IP to startups who raise significant VC or angel (VC/A) financing.

The program funds up to 5–8 projects per year for an average of $100,000 each. Each project must involve a collaboration between UM faculty from any College of Engineering department and from a medical clinical department. Each project aims to generate a new medical device, surgical tool, or clinical diagnostic test. Project teams are mentored by a team of experienced industry experts to guide projects to the point of licensing the intellectual property into a start-up company that goes on to raise funding from VCs/As or licensing the intellectual property to an existing revenue-generating company.

Funding for the program began in 2006 in the form of annual $1 million grants, and evolved to an endowment agreement for the $20 million in 2011. In addition to UM, the WHCF has awarded grants or endowments to 15 other universities (Fig. 12.5) that have created Coulter programs at their respective universities. While each program has subtle differences in organizational structure, they all share a common theme of utilizing an industry-based approach and process to generate follow on funding through VC/A investments or licensing to industry.

Boston University	University of Louisville
Case Western Reserve University*	University of Miami
Columbia University	University of Michigan*
Drexel University*	University of Missouri
Duke University*	University of Pittsburgh
Georgia Institute of Technology*	University of So. California
Johns Hopkins University	University of Virginia*
Stanford University*	University of Washington

*WHCF Endowed Programs

Fig. 12.5 Coulter-Funded Programs in the United States

Operational efforts for each program are led by a Coulter Program Director (CPD) and the Biomedical Engineering Chair serving as the Program Principal Investigator (PI). Each program has Assistant CPDs or Project Managers to support the efforts of the CPD. The collective group of CPDs meet on a periodic basis to share best practices, host an annual investment forum, and meet with business development representatives from medical device companies creating tremendous synergies across programs. With common goals, the Coulter teams from the different universities with Coulter funding have established a strong community where they have been able to leverage education, networking, and connections to enhance opportunities for reaching follow-on funding and industry licensing goals.

Additionally, each program is overseen by an Oversight Committee (OC), who have fiduciary responsibility for programs, conduct project reviews and make project selection and funding decisions. OCs play a strong role in providing guidance and direction to project teams, and are instrumental in making industry connections. At each university, OCs are comprised of VC/A investors, medical device and diagnostics business development directors and VP level representatives, Office of Technology Transfer directors, serial entrepreneurs in the medical device space, senior clinical representatives from the medical school, regulatory strategy experts, the BME Chair, and often other BME faculty. A key differentiator for Coulter programs is the active project management approach and focus on providing business leadership alongside technical and clinical expertise. The main value of the program are the resources and expertise provided to support new product planning and early stage medical technology product development efforts. The funding is of secondary importance.

Coulter Commercialization Process and Funding Cycle

Each Coulter program follows generally the same process, which is modeled based on industry best practices for evaluating opportunities and creating a milestone-based

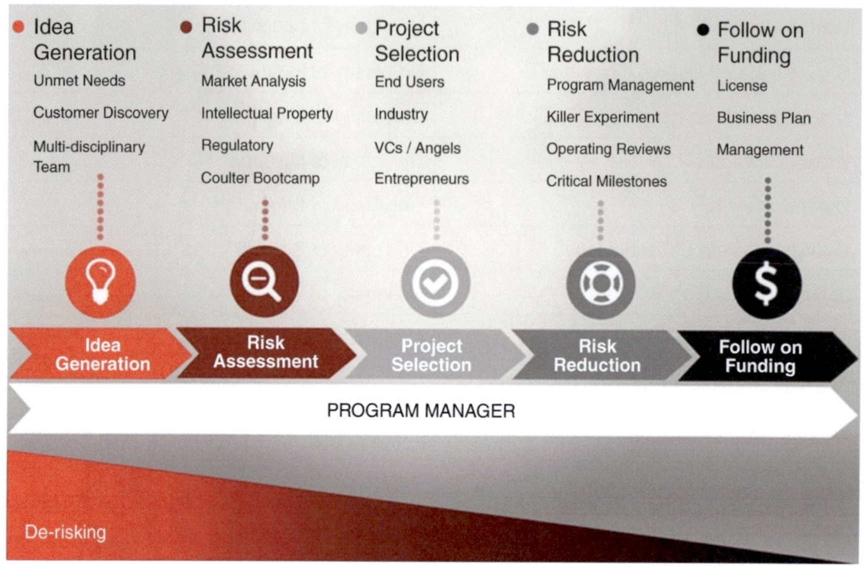

Fig. 12.6 Creating a milestone-based funding approach to reduce risk and lead to licenses. Source: WHCF

funding approach to reduce risk and lead to licenses to industry or VC/A follow on funding. (Fig. 12.6) This process involves a significant level of review and evaluation prior to project selection and funding. The oversight committee tends to focus an eye towards identifying a "killer experiment" or proof of concept demonstration that will significantly increase the value if successful, or demonstrate lack of medical or commercial viability if unsuccessful. Killer experiments, business development goals and early stage product development become a large focus of funding efforts and milestones.

Coulter Model: Proven Success for over 12 Years

The Coulter process has proven successful in addressing many of the challenges with moving academic medical innovations into well-funded companies to complete commercialization. According to WHCF, from July 2006 through December 2017, combined Coulter university efforts across all 16 Coulter programs has resulted in:

- 661 projects funded for a total of $173.5 million in funding
- 192 projects (29%) resulted in VC/A backed startups or licenses to industry

    - 135 VC/A funded startups
    - 57 Licenses to industry

Nearly one out of three funded projects translated into a VC/A backed startup or license to industry. Of note, projects culminating in additional government grants only (i.e. NIH, DOD, NSF, SBIR, STTR, etc.) were not counted as exits. The rationale being that VC backed financing or licensing to a strategic provides greater commercial validation and probability of successfully reaching the market through adequately financed and resourced commercial entities. As VCs report funding only 1% of potential opportunities considered [3], we believe that employing the Coulter process greatly increases the probability of translating academic surgical and other medical innovations into professionally financed companies or license agreements with strategics.

Evolution of Best Practices - the Michigan Coulter Story

The University of Michigan Coulter program (UM-CP) has experienced similar success over this time period. UM-CP funding began in 2006. For projects with first year of funding between 2006 and 2017:

- 50 projects were funded for a total of $8.1 million in funding
- 12 projects (24%) resulted in VC/A backed startups or licenses to industry

  - 8 VC/A funded startups
  - 4 Licenses to industry (strategics)

However, when evaluating outcomes over different time periods, we see the impact of challenges to commercializing medical and surgical innovations, and a strategic approach taken by the UM-CP to overcome these challenges.

Early Success, but Lull Period after Endowment

Between 2006 and 2010, the UM-CP was funded through annual $1 M grants from the WHCF, and was one of the early medical translational research funding programs at UM. In this time period, UM-CP funded 19 projects and generated five exits, all start-ups, that each raised VC or Angel financing. This constituted a 26% exit rate. Successful startups emanating out of UM-CP funding during this time frame include Histosonics (http://www.histosonics.com) who raised $11 million in 2009 and Tissue Regeneration Systems (https://www.tissuesys.com) who raised $2 million by 2010. Histosonics is developing a non-invasive focused ultrasound platform for targeted tissue ablation, while TRS creates patient specific bioresorbable scaffolds and bone implants. This period is referred to as the Pre-Endowment period.

The UM-CP received the endowment from the WHCF in 2011, which started the first 5-year time period where the program was evaluated based on exit metrics. From 2011 to 2014, while excluding one project that took a different approach that will be described later, 14 projects were funded with only two reaching the exit stage with angel backed startups for a 14% exit rate.

Arguably the decline in exits during this period coincided with the economic downturn and the decline in VC investments in med tech companies. Series A investment as a percent of total VC investments in medtech declined from 19% in 2006 to 10% in 2016 [2]. Series A investments are the initial funding rounds for medtech companies, and typically occur after startups raise smaller amounts of funding from other sources. In the Deloitte report, a business development executive from a large medtech company noted that "early-stage companies might put lots of weight on building clinical evidence but relatively less on areas of importance to strategic buyers, such as ability to build manufacturing scale, reimbursement, and a compelling economic value proposition." With the decline in VC funding, meeting strategic buyer expectations while projects are still in the academic setting has proven to be critically important to translating academic medical innovations into commercial entities.

During the time period from 2011 to 2014, UM-CP project selection and management focused on killer experiments and risk reduction with little up-front due diligence to guide project selection and little product development work to meet strategic buyer-needs during funding. We refer to this period as the Risk-Reduction Focus period (Fig. 12.7). In this Risk-Reduction period, commercial viability was presumed based on clinical faculty perceptions, cursory reviews of secondary data sources and, internal feedback from the OC. Most of the focus of efforts for projects awarded during this time period was on technical risk reduction with "Killer experiments" testing the viability of technology that would be incorporated into the envisioned product. This was intended to demonstrate proof of concept. However, many of the projects involved product concepts that required long development time horizons with multiple killer experiments. The culmination of funding often provided demonstration of some level of technical performance, but did not lead to investible product concepts ready for investors. In most cases, a well-developed roadmap to an exit with confirmation of interest from target strategics or VC investors was not developed prior to funding. When presented to VCs and strategics, most of these projects were considered "too early" after Coulter funding.

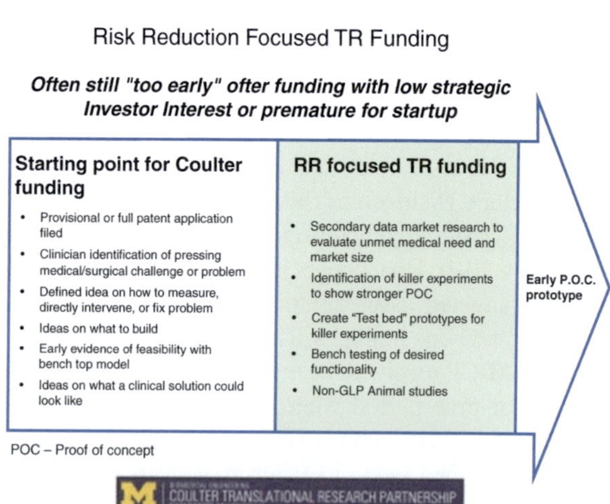

Fig. 12.7 Source: University of Michigan Coulter Program

However, one funded project stood out as an exception that helped set the stage for future UM-CP projects. In 2013, UM-CP began funding for a project to develop a novel means of interfacing with peripheral nerves to capture nerve signals at the fascicle level, digitize signals and use these signals to control advanced prosthetic robotic upper limbs in upper limb amputees. UM Professor of Plastic Surgery Paul Cederna developed a surgical procedure to harvest and deploy small muscle grafts as sheaths wrapped around the end of severed nerves. Each muscle wrap created a mini-bioamplifier for nerve signals that could be transmitted to electrodes and used to provide fine motor control of robotic limbs. This harvested muscle nerve wrap (regenerative peripheral nerve interface or RPNI) regenerated and created an effective means for amplifying nerve signals. Observations of RPNIs created during small animal studies revealed that none of the RPNIs led to neuroma development. Cederna later performed this procedure on amputee patients with refractory neuroma pain and discovered that the RPNIs prevented neuroma redevelopment and eliminated neuroma-related pain in most patients. Each surgical RPNI placement took up to 45 min to perform.

In 2014, Coulter and the UM Office of Technology Transfer commissioned primary market research with clinicians across multiple specialties and payers to assess perceptions of neuroma related unmet medical needs and gauge reactions to a target product profile of a device concept that could automate the RPNI procedure. The significant level of unmet need was confirmed, and the device concept was found compelling amongst surgeons, if the procedure provided durable results. Based on the strong clinical findings and positive perception of the device concept, UM-Coulter in 2014 funded the development of a device with the goal of automating the procedure and reducing surgical time to a target goal of 10 min per RPNI. Funding for work on advanced prosthetic limb control with RPNIs continued, and the neuroma funding was carved out as a separate project.

Dr. Cederna partnered with Mechanical Engineering Professor Albert Shih, PhD, and PhD-candidate Jeffrey Plott, and student Jordan Kreda to develop multiple prototype iterations, each one striving towards target goals of safely facilitating the procedure and reducing procedure time. After multiple iterations, the team successfully met this goal with a prototype design that worked well in bench testing and early studies in a pig model (Fig. 12.8). Along with the Coulter team and working with the UM Tech Transfer team, a mid-sized medical device company in the biopsy tool space was identified and approached to explore interest in licensing. The company was invited to UM for an overview presentation of the device concept where the team shared plans for a large animal study to demonstrate device performance. We were able to generate early interest and confirmation that the research plan under Coulter funding would justify licensing, pending successful outcomes. The company also required confirmation of an FDA designation as a Class II device with minimal clinical requirements prior to licensing. To address the regulatory question, Coulter commissioned and worked closely with MethodSense, Inc. (http://methodsense.com/), a regulatory strategy firm based in Morrisville, NC, to prepare for and lead discussions with FDA in an FDA pre-submission meeting to

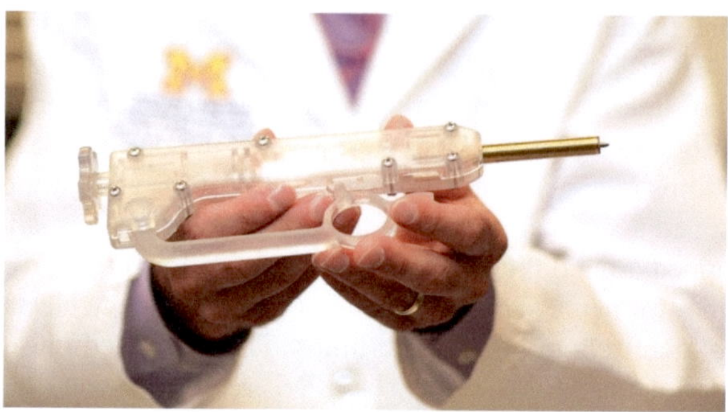

Fig. 12.8 Source: UM Coulter website. "Coulter Program funding supported the development of this surgical tool held by U-M Professor of Plastic Surgery Paul Cederna, MD. He and his U-M Plastic Surgery colleagues, along with U-M Mechanical Engineering Professor Albert Shih, PhD, PhD-candidate Jeffrey Plott, and student Jordan Kreda, developed the tool to facilitate surgery for treating painful neuromas. The surgical tool was licensed to RLS Interventional in March 2016." Photo: Chris Stranad

gain an understanding of FDA expectations. These efforts ultimately led to a license agreement in 2016, and this device is still in development as of the writing of this article.

Key takeaways: Blindly focusing on a "killer experiment" (experiment to demonstrate technical de-risking or early evidence of device performance) alone is not sufficient in most cases to generate investor or strategics interest. However, by proactively searching for a strategic investor and structuring milestones and funding plans to support a potential deal, academic funding programs can constructively collaborate with strategics prior to any licensing arrangements to improve odds of licensing and accelerate commercialization through a strategic partner. Starting in 2015, UM-CP instituted program changes to meet these goals. These program changes also led to an increased focus on meeting investment criteria for strategics, with the realization that meeting these goals also improves opportunities for raising VC funding if the exit goal is company formation.

Evolution of the Michigan Coulter Program

Early Due Diligence/Strategic Planning: The C3i Program

In 2014, the WHCF embarked on a business development and strategic planning program they named Coulter College Commercializing Innovation or "C3i" program. This program was funded through a National Institute of Biomedical Imaging and Bioengineering NIH division grant for a select number of SBIR Phase I awardees to support their efforts with business planning and pitch development for investors. The program involved a high level of mentoring and guidance over a series of weekly conference call meetings culminating in a 3-day boot camp where teams

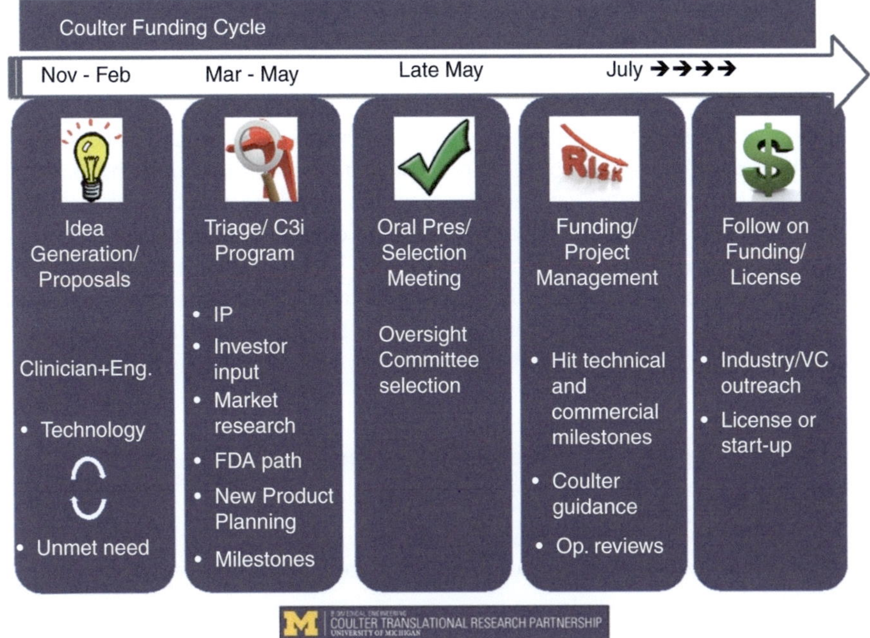

Fig. 12.9 Source: University of Michigan Coulter Program

polished investor pitches and participated in an investor pitch competition. CPDs from the different Coulter universities served as project managers and mentors for company teams in the program, while industry business advisors were engaged to provide additional mentoring support.

In 2015, the UM-CP adopted this program and customized the approach and curriculum to fit Michigan program needs for improving project selection, and providing business development support for project teams seeking Coulter funding. The funding cycle was structured to incorporate C3i as part of a stage-gate funding cycle process. Following a triage step to screen project proposals, project teams are selected for C3i. C3i is run over a two-month time period leading up to a final selection meeting where teams pitch the Coulter OC who select projects for funding (Fig. 12.9).

The real value of C3i is the process of transitioning from a research mindset to one of new product planning and business development. The objective of the Michigan C3i Program is to help Coulter proposal applicants build their full proposal and pitch deck, as well as answer three fundamental questions:

1. **Does their envisioned product address a true unmet clinical need that health care providers and payors are willing to solve?**
2. **Is there a viable business opportunity?**
3. **Will the proposed research de-risk the project to the point of generating investor or industry interest in the product concept?**

C3i is designed to provide Coulter Proposal Teams with the specialized business frameworks and essential tools for successful translation of biomedical technologies from lab to market.

Teams are guided through a series of interactive exercises, and benefit from expert biomedical consulting firms who conduct primary market research, competitive landscape assessments, and regulatory roadmaps to pressure-test the commercial viability of envisioned product concepts and explore the unique requirements for product development and commercialization. Teams also work with medical device industry mentor expert advisors, investors, and outside consultants who provide insights into the market sector, new product planning, IP, regulatory, and reimbursement requirements specific for their projects.

As part of C3i, The Michigan Coulter program invests up to $15,000 to support the commercial planning for each project. Investments include hiring external experts to complete one or more of the following:

- Competitive landscape assessment
- Primary market research interviews with target audiences for envisioned product
- Regulatory roadmaps
- IP landscape assessments
- Reimbursement assessments

C3i Process and Timing

The C3i program is structured into three sections to validate the need, validate the business opportunity, and then package the opportunity with a milestone driven research and business development plan the team pitches to the Coulter OC for funding (Fig. 12.10). The end goal is to generate Coulter funding milestones to increase value and the probability of reaching an exit.

In this process, teams refine their target product profiles, and milestone plans while preparing for their Coulter presentations at the selection meeting through a series of weekly "home work" deliverables and information gleaned from mentors, market analysis, regulatory reviews, and market research interviews with key stakeholders. Deliverables are designed as commercialization planning exercises that follow industry standards in new product planning and development. Teams present findings from assignments at the start of each weekly team meeting, during which time coaches, and industry/OC mentors provide feedback.

The final deliverables of the C3i program is a Blueprint report providing a foundation for new product planning and justification for research milestones the team is requesting Coulter to fund, along with a 15-min pitch deck for use during the Selection meeting presentation. The Blueprint report (Fig. 12.11) provides a frame-

Fig. 12.10 Source: University of Michigan Coulter Program

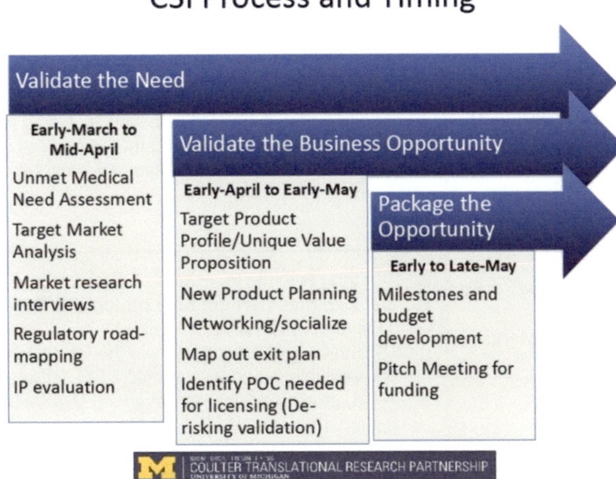

Project Summary

Project Title	Automated Detection and Labeling of High Frequency Osci llations (HFO) in Clinical EEG systems
Investigators	William Stacey, MD (Neurology, Biomedical Engineering); Stephen Gliske, PhD (Neurology, Biomedical Engineering)
Technology area	Medical Software
Target therapeutic area	Refractory epilepsy
Brief "One line" Description of Research	Clinical validation of the automated labeling of HFO markings by independent reviewers and assessing the clinical utility of HFOs for guiding surgical decision making.
Product type to be developed	Add-on software module containing an algorithm for automated HFO detection which can be integrated into existing EEG platforms.
Expected application or indication for new product	Identification of HFOs within EEG tracings to aid in pre-surgical planning in refractory epilepsy patients. HFOs have great potential to identify seizure networks faster and with greater precision than the current methods of using traditional low-resolution data such as seizure spike detection software or manually reviewing EEG traces.
Stage	Prototyping: Developing code to allow t he software to integrate with commercial EEG software systems.
Primary funding source	NIH R01, NIH K01
Other funding	Doris Duke Charitable Foundation
Total funding amount supporting research	$385,000/year 2017-2018; $235,000/ year 2019-2020 (includes other related projects)
IP Status	US Patent Application xxxx, awaiting first office action. Converted to a full US utility patent.
Company formation status	Pre-company
University Licensing status	No option
Business Strategy Goal	License to existing companies in EEG market: xxx, xxx, xxx

Fig. 12.11 Sample Blueprint Report (full research milestones not shown)

Where To Play – Target Market/ Problem To Be Solved

Description of Ideal target customer	Target customers Include: 1) the clinicians who review EEG for epilepsy surgery planning (the end users), and 2) the companies making EEG software used by these clinicians, i.e. Natus, Persyst, cadwell, Nihon Kohden.
Target Market Size	• The total revenue for Persyst (EEG viewing software) was $3M in 2016. • The total revenue from EEG device and systems for Natus (Neurodiagnostics company) in 2016 was $168.2 M. • 181 Level·4 epilepsy centers in the US (NAEC), each with 3·15 epileptologists, and with 10·100 EEG software licenses. • In US, there are 1 million patients with medication resistant epilepsy who require intra-cranial EEG monitoring.
Current "Gold Standard"	Visual interpretation of EEG traces by epileptologists at low resolution (< 40 Hz). This method completely ignores HFO detections. HFOs are the most promising biomarker to improve efficacy of epilepsy surgery, with many publications in high-level journals for 15 years. Although the newest acquisition systems are capable of recording HFOs, no software exists to automatically detect and visualize HFOs in the EEG context. HFOs remain completely unutilized clinically.

How to Win – What will product profile need to look like to generate adoption and sustained use?

Target Unique Value Proposition	For patients with refractory epilepsy, this software provides the only commercial program capable of automatically labeling HFO events within EEG viewins software, thereby providing a novel source of data for neurosurgeons to improve surgical decision making and potentially increasing the success rate for resection surgeries to reduce seizure frequency or provide seizure freedom and reduce the amount of brain tissue removed during surgery.	
Target Product profile (TPP)	Description	An add-on software module which integrates with existing EEG acquisition software that automatically generates HFO labels, identifying the location of the HFOs and characterizing whether they are likely to be pathological.
	Efficacy/Performance	HFO labels have sensitivity/specificity and kappa scores that are indistinguishable from the variability among human reviewers (85%/85%). Labels generated prior to review by clinicians, either in real time or within 4 hours after closing a study.
	Safety/Tolerability	The product does not interact with the patient and the data generated by the product is being interpreted by physicians. Therefore, there are no safety risks or tolerability issues with this product.
	Convenience/Ease of Use/ Efficiency Improvement	Require no more than 15% increase in the amount of time needed to review an EEG study. Allow clinicians to visualize when/where HFOs occur without requiring them to filter and recalibrate the viewer.
Clinical Regulatory Strategy	Expecting FDA Class II with 510(k) submission	
Anticipated Business Model	License software to existing EEG companies to be Integrated into their future product lines.	

Team # 1 | HFOs for EEG

Fig. 12.11 (continued)

How to Get There – Research Milestones

Research Milestones	Objectives	Success Criteria
AIM 1: Interface HFO detector software within Persyst and Natus software	Get a working prototype with Natus and Penyst	Ability to show HFO detections within clinical EEG in Natus Neuroworks and Persyst Insight acquisition software programs.
Ajm 1.1: Hire a computer programmer skilled in developing prototype software	Develop required coding specifications, verification and validation procedures for integrating HFO detection algorithm within existing FDA approved EEG software. Hire programmer with appropriate skill set to code and perform V&V.	Hire a programmer before 7/1/17 with the required backeround/skills under a work for hire agreement. Programmer must be skilled in C++, have experience integrating software, meeting national regulatory standards, and collaborating with commercial entities
Aim 1.2: Write code to intesrate algorithm with commercial EEG systems	Complete development of a C++ program that includes our alsorithm and allows bidirectional dataflow with the clinical software.	Completion of all required code writing, debugging, and verification. The software program will read and process data in < 4 hours per 24 hour record.
Aim 1.3: Validate use case	Ensure C++ program provides simple user experience to accomplish product goals	Files with HFO markings will open using clinical versions of Natus Neuroworks and Persyst Insight. Markings will be visible with standard clinical protocols.

Team # 1 | HFOs for EEG

Fig. 12.11 (continued)

work to define the envisioned product emanating out of Coulter funding. These reports are structured to address the three key questions for new product planning:

- Where to play – Target market/problem to be solved
- How to win – What will the product need to look like to generate adoption and sustained use
- How to get there – Research milestones

Next Phase Evolution – Academic Research to Early Product Development

In addition to utilization of C3i for project due diligence and strategic planning, the UM-CP team came to the realization that to generate investor interest, better "hand-off" packages were required to meet investor expectations. Whether a startup or strategic, companies have defined processes for medical device product development and a keen eye towards "time to market" when evaluating new product opportunities. The extent to which academic innovations can exit universities further down the product development continuum, the higher the probability of generating serious interest from strategics or other investors.

Medical device development can be broken up into two general stages; Design and Go-to-market (Fig. 12.12). Since 2015, UM-CP projects have looked to move beyond risk reduction with "killer experiments" to incorporate more Design stages of development. Go-to-market related activities are beyond what can be accomplished in an academic setting.

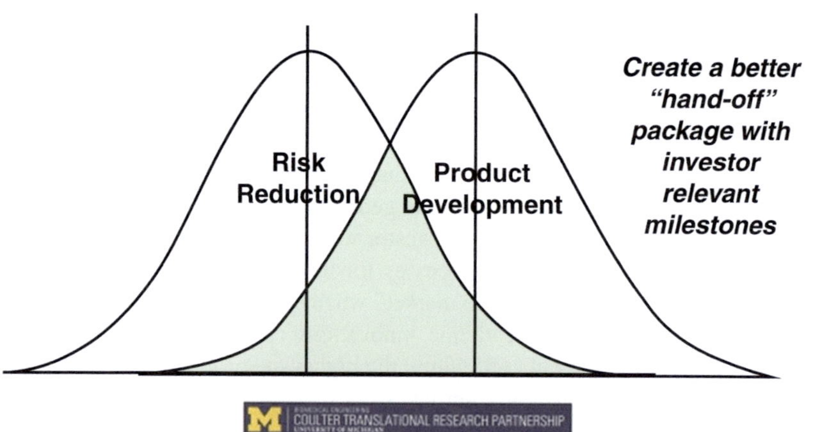

Fig. 12.12 Source: University of Michigan Coulter Program

Recent UM-CP projects have incorporated Design related milestones including:

- Outsourcing development to medical device design shops to build advanced prototypes
- Initiating design control documentation and building a device under design controls
- Submitting an Investigational Device Exemption (IDE) application for a first in human study for an implantable device.

Recent projects have also had a greater focus on interacting with FDA through the Q-Submission process, with multiple product concepts emanating out of Coulter funding receiving risk designations or confirmation of planned regulatory approach. As mentioned with the NeuromaTool project, determining the level of clinical performance requirements was instrumental in reaching a licensing deal. By engaging in the concepts of risk assessments and design controls, more focus has been placed on designing product concepts to mitigate risks and develop design specification requirements for the ultimate product. As such, the grant focus of continuous innovation has slowly been replaced with the notion of "locking down" on a viable product concept.

Engaging with project teams throughout the C3i process and focusing on product development milestones has required a partnering approach with project teams where the Coulter team has become an active partner. Through networking and effectively contracting with external consultants and vendors, Coulter funded project teams have realized significant value and service beyond the actual funding itself (Fig. 12.13).

UM Coulter Value Beyond Money

Active partnership with comprehensive resources

Market assessments	New product development planning and costing
Primary market research	Design control development
Market/ Demand forecast modeling	Design reviews
Project planning/milestone setting	Risk assessments
Vendor scouting	FDA pre-sub meeting dossier prep
Vendor negotiations and hiring	FDA submissions
Investor scouting and outreach	FDA meetings
Pitch deck development	Working with design and mfg cos. for prototype development
Investor meeting planning	Animal study designs
Input on deal terms	Human clinical trial designs

Highly networked within UM ecosystem and beyond:

- **UM:** Med School, COE, Tech Transfer, FFMI, MICHR, MCIRCC, TBI Fund, GI Innovations Fund, MTRAC, Monroe Brown Fund, Surgery Innovation Fund,
- **External:** OC interactions, C3i industry and investor mentors, Coulter Foundation, 16 Coulter schools, AA Spark, Mich Bio, MEDC, Regulatory strategy firms, Med device design and manufacturing firms

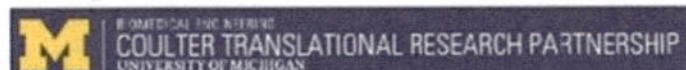

Fig. 12.13 Source: University of Michigan Coulter Program

Results of UM-CP Evolution: Recent Success 2015–2017: New Product Planning and Development Focus Period

For projects with first year of funding between 2015 and 2017 with the inclusion of the neuroma tool project:

- 16 projects were funded
- As of the end of 2018, 5 projects (31%) resulted in VC/A backed startups or licenses to industry

  - 1 VC/A funded startups
  - 4 Licenses to industry (strategics)

As such, the evolution of the UM-CP appears to be making an impact with a 31% exit rate for UM Coulter projects funded between 2015 and 2017, vs. a 14% exit rate over the prior 4-year Risk Reduction time period. As of December 2018, two additional projects are poised for near term exits; one is in due diligence with an investor group interested in forming a company around a Coulter funded technology, and another project is at the approved IDE stage and about to start a first-in-human pilot study. This project has an interested strategic partner who have provided significant development support and have indicated they will pursue licensing if results are positive. If these two additional projects exit, the exit rate would reach nearly 44% for projects funded during this more recent time period.

Recent UM-CP efforts have focused on licensing to a strategic with 4 out of 5 exits as industry licenses. Company formation has been a fallback option or option to pursue if inventors wish to pursue this route. However, identification of viable management teams and raising venture financing remain a significant challenge. Fortunately, venture capital financing has increased over the past year with emphasis on digital health wearable device funding [6]. This may reinvigorate future efforts with company formation and VC/A fund raising.

Success Stories

Exits during the 2015–2017 time period provide demonstrations of successful execution of the New Product Planning and Development strategy as illustrated by the following three projects that led to licensing deals with strategics, and one project well positioned for an exit that has reached the IDE and clinical trial stage.

Arterial Everter Project (2015 Funding)

This project involved the development of an accessory for an FDA cleared device on the market, the GEM™ Microvascular Anastomotic Coupler from Synovis Micro Companies Alliance, a Baxter subsidiary. The GEM coupler device (Fig. 12.14) is

Fig. 12.14 http://bme.
umich.edu/
a-better-way-to-connect-
arteries/

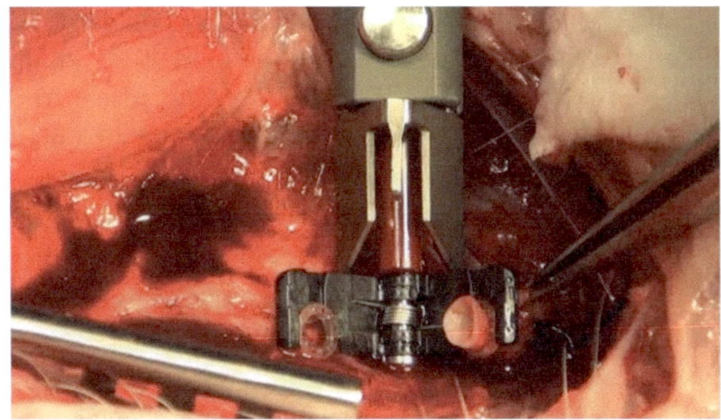

used during reconstructive surgery to connect blood vessels, and works well for connecting veins, but is extremely challenging to couple arteries. The arterial everter developed in this project enables the GEM Coupler device to couple arteries as well as veins. Hence the everter stood to nearly double the market for the GEM Coupler as both arteries and veins need to be connected during reconstructive procedures. This project emanated out of a student design project and was at the early concept stage prior to Coulter funding. Coulter provided funding to complete design work and test in an animal model. Coulter worked with the clinician and engineering project team to engage with Synovis and Baxter to confirm their commercial interest and design a pilot large animal study with input from both UM clinicians and Baxter. Baxter and Synovis representatives travelled to UM to observe the study and were able to directly observe arterial coupling with the everter. After generating positive outcomes, the UM Tech Transfer licensing team successfully negotiated a licensing agreement [8, 9]. Throughout this project frequent communications with Synovis and Baxter confirmed licensing interest prior to funding and ensured that the research plan was sufficient to convince Baxter to license and take over development of the Everter. Although UM assumed all risks in development for a device with limited exit options, the relationships and trust built over the course of the project facilitated the Baxter due diligence process and licensing negotiations with the UM Tech Transfer licensing team.

HFO Project: Automated Detection and Labeling of High Frequency Oscillations (HFOs) in Clinical EEG Systems (2017 Funding):

This project involved software development to detect HFOs from within EEG viewing software. See Fig. 12.11 Sample Blueprint report for project details. For patients with refractory epilepsy, this software provides the ability to automatically label HFO events within EEG viewing software, thereby providing a novel source of data for study as a biomarker to help locate seizure loci and improve surgical decision making for resection surgeries to reduce seizure frequency.

Based on primary market research with epileptologists, this project was still considered at the research stage, and the market was dominated by a small number of players in the EEG recording and viewing space. At first glance, this project was considered too early for funding and too small of a market. However, with guidance from Coulter and medical device industry business development mentors, the clinical PI on the project was able to reach out to the CEOs of leading industry players in this space to set up meetings where we were able to gauge interest. CEOs or senior management from three EEG companies confirmed a very high level of commercial interest, and frustration with the inability to automate HFO detection. They also provided an indication of the level of verification testing and validation that they would need to see before considering licensing.

Three key milestones were identified as requirements these companies would need to see before licensing. Interface HFO detector code with an EEG company clinical software, develop a viable methodology and test for quantification of HFO detection sensitivity and specificity, and demonstrate clinical utility based on a survey with other epileptologists. Coulter funded these milestones. Milestones were completed and met target success criteria. In November, 2018, a licensing agreement was signed with one of the EEG recording and software companies. This project provided an example of seeking to understand industry needs, capitalizing on momentum to help a company reach a strategic goal, and identification of strategics' licensing requirements. Note: Due to proprietary reasons, the company name is not being disclosed at this time.

Slit Stent II:

Epiphora, or severe tearing, is often caused by lacrimal duct blockage and can lead to both swelling and infections. Treatment includes a surgical DCR procedure to create new opening to allow tear drainage. Lacrimal stents are used to facilitate healing, but do not drain tears. Patients continue to experience Epiphora symptoms for months post-surgery. A UM team lead by an oculoplastic surgeon and mechanical engineering researcher designed a stent to allow for drainage of tears to provide immediate symptom relief.

Coulter provided funding for Slit Stent design iterations, facilitated a partnership with a leading manufacturer of lacrimal stents, and helped secure an FDA Investigational Device Exemption (IDE) for the Slit-Stent device. These devices will be used in a UM-sponsored, 15-patient clinical trial at the UM Kellogg Eye Center starting in early 2019 [1].

This project was unique in that the Slit Stent II device is an implantable device for greater than 28 days, which requires an IDE. The project team was able to partner with a leading lacrimal stent company to use their existing FDA approved stent as a starting point for the manufacture of Slit Stent II. This avoided many of the costs that would have been required if the team developed a totally new stent (i.e. medical grade material sourcing, bio-compatibility testing, mechanical testing, packaging and sterilization protocol development and validation). These costs would be beyond the scope of typical university funding.

Coulter worked with UM Tech Transfer to secure an agreement with the company to provide stents free of charge, reference their FDA documentation related to their stent used in Slit Stent II manufacturing, and to provide multiple in-kind services including packaging and sterilization using their validated sterilization process, and mechanical testing all in exchange for right of first negotiation or first look at the data from the clinical study. Thus, for no monetary cost, the team was able to avoid significant development costs and a much longer development timeline by co-developing the device with a strategic partner. This project also required the development of design controls related to the Slit Stent II device manufacturing. This makes UM the manufacturer of record for the device and the device will be very close to the FDA submission stage after completion of the clinical study. With such a high level of coordination with a strategic and advanced development of the product, this project will move directly into licensing negotiations if the clinical study shows a successful outcome.

Summary and Conclusion

By employing a systematic approach for both project selection and determination of investor relevant milestones, academic translational research funding programs can improve probabilities of achieving exits to commercial partners and accelerate commercialization of medical and surgical innovations. This approach requires a keen awareness of potential exit pathways and the milestone requirements commercial entities will expect prior to licensing medical technologies out of academia. With early and often interactions with investors, and leveraging networks and available academic medical center funding resources, these goals are often achievable. As demonstrated by our Coulter Translational Research Partnership program between the medical school and the engineering school, executing on these milestones has led to an increase in exits to both strategics and startups who successfully go on to raise venture or angel capital financing.

References

1. Clinicaltrials.gov Identifier: NCT03705000. Safety and Efficacy of the Slit Stent II Lacrimal Stent for the Treatment of Nasolacrimal Duct Obstruction. 2018. https://clinicaltrials.gov/ct2/show/NCT03705000?term=slit+stent+II&rank=1.
2. Deloitte. Out of the valley of death. How can entrepreneurs, corporations, and investors reinvigorate eary-stage medtech innovation? 2017.
3. Gompers. How do venture capitalists make decisions? Working paper no. 22587. National Bureau of economic research, 2016.

4. Makower J, et al. FDA impact on US Medical technology innovation: Stanford University; 2010.
5. Pienta KJ. Successfully accelerating translational research at an Academic Medical Center: the University of Michigan-Coulter Translational Research Partnership Program. Clin Transl Sci. 2010;3(6):316–8.
6. Shah S. Early-stage medtech venture investment is up, driven by digitally enabled diagnostics. But is the market ready? In: Deloitte; 2018.
7. SVP. Healthcare investments and exits report 2018. In: Silicon Valley Bank; 2018. https://www.svb.com/healthcare-investments-exits-report/.
8. University of Michigan. A Better Way to Connect Arteries. 2018a.
9. University of Michigan. National Institutes of Health: Supporting Research at Michigan. 2018b.
10. Wikipedia/Translational Research. https://en.wikipedia.org/wiki/Translational_research

Chapter 13
Creating a Multidisciplinary Surgical Innovations Group at an Academic Medical Center to Stimulate Surgery Faculty Technology Development

Veeshal H. Patel, Michael R. Harrison, Elizabeth A. Gress, Shuvo Roy, Prashant Chopra, Stacy S. Kim, and Hanmin Lee

Section 1: Academic Institutions with Surgical "Innovations Programs"

As surgery has evolved, a number of academic institutions have provided resources in order to establish innovations programs for their faculty. Surgical departments, in particular, have been early adopters of this concept. We believe this is due to the nature of the work and scope of the surgeon; as masters of anatomy and physiology, surgeons are well placed in the medical device space to create new tools and make iterative evolutionary modifications to existing technologies to improve myriad issues experienced in their clinical practice.

While this chapter focuses largely on the Surgical Innovations program at the University of California, San Francisco, there are a number of forward-thinking initiatives that have arisen from academic surgical departments nationwide. These include the Byers Center for Biodesign at Stanford University, University of Michigan Surgical Innovations program, Dartmouth-Hitchcock Center for Surgical Innovation, Harvard/MIT/BU Consortia for Improving Medicine with Innovation and Technology (CIMIT), and Texas Medical Center Biodesign program. Each program has followed a unique development pathway in the context of their own departments, universities, and industry collaborations, but one thing rings true across the spectrum: academic surgeons are driving innovation and the development of new technologies through their institutions.

V. H. Patel · M. R. Harrison · E. A. Gress · S. Roy · P. Chopra · S. S. Kim · H. Lee (✉)
Division of Pediatric Surgery, Department of Surgery, University of California,
San Francisco, CA, USA
e-mail: vhpatel@uw.edu; michael.harrison@ucsf.edu; elizabeth.gress@ucsf.edu; shuvo.roy@ucsf.edu; prashant.copra@ucsf.edu; stacy.kim@ucsf.edu; hanmin.lee@ucsf.edu

© Springer Nature Switzerland AG 2019
M. S. Cohen, L. Kao (eds.), *Success in Academic Surgery: Innovation and Entrepreneurship*, Success in Academic Surgery,
https://doi.org/10.1007/978-3-030-18613-5_13

Section 2: History and Roadmap of Creating an Academic Surgical Innovations Group at UCSF

The creation of an academic surgical innovations ecosystem at the University of California, San Francisco, began in the Department of Surgery 12 years ago, in 2006. A group of like-minded surgeons, including Dr. Michael Harrison, Dr. Marshall Stoller, Dr. Quan Duh, and Dr. Hanmin Lee, began meeting each week before Surgery Grand Rounds in order to brainstorm and develop technical solutions for clinical problems. All had been experienced surgeon innovators. Notably, Dr. Harrison is widely regarded as the father of fetal surgery, having identified the clinical need that without intervention, some fetuses would not survive. The clinical and research initiatives from this clinical need resulted in the creation of many specific tools for fetal surgery, from staplers and endoscopic equipment to specialized catheters and fetal monitoring systems. Another noted innovator in this early innovator club, Dr. Marshall Stoller, is a Urologist at UCSF. His group created a novel device and disruptive technical alternative to standard shockwave lithotripsy, which is currently in clinical trials in India.

The most widely adopted successes come in the realm of fetal surgery, led by Dr. Michael Harrison, prior to the creation of the collaborative group mentioned above. Dr. Harrison and his team began the field, created the tools, and refined the technical nuances needed to enable safe surgery in a fetus. They continue to create new devices and disease targets, continually advancing existing procedures. From the first open fetal surgeries in 1983, to the advent of minimally invasive fetal techniques and the creation of the ex utero intrapartum treatment (EXIT) procedure for fetal delivery in 1995, to multicenter clinical trials in 2002, Dr. Harrison and his teams have succeeded in laying the framework needed for wider adoption and further trials for fetal interventions. The fetal surgery story is a precursor to the future Surgical Innovations group: what began as a weekly meeting amongst like-minded, motivated physicians grew gradually into an expansive center spurred by the hopes of clinical impact permitted by technological innovation.

As this model continued to evolve into the group that began to convene in 2006, the surgeons' scope expanded to adult devices and numerous clinical applications. Initially, engineering talent was contracted using engineering firms in the greater San Francisco Bay Area. Over years, the early morning meetings of this innovators club expanded further, resulting in an influx of surgical residents and trainees participating in the process, and the creation of a more formal team with internally employed engineers, consisting largely of biomedical engineers, mechanical engineers, and electrical engineers. The program was also spurred by partnerships with the University of California, Berkeley, and local design and manufacturing engineering firms. These firms assisted in product design, prototyping, and testing to help scale the initiatives that initially came from the aforementioned weekly brainstorms.

In 2009, a unique opportunity to further develop the ecosystem presented itself through the Food & Drug Administration's (FDA) Pediatric Device Consortia (PDC) program, established under a Congressional mandate. Administered by the Office for Orphan Products Development, the program was charged with facilitating the development, production, and distribution of pediatric medical devices and either resulting in, or substantially contributing to, market approval of medical devices designed specifically for use in children. As such, UCSF was one of the inaugural four grantees of this award. This funding established the program's infrastructure, which led to hiring additional in-house engineers and creating a formal engine for surgical residents to participate in the various projects during their academic research years. In addition to this grant, Dr. Shuvo Roy was recruited to UCSF from the Cleveland Clinic to lead numerous initiatives in the Department of Bioengineering and Therapeutic Sciences, including his landmark Artificial Kidney Project. With a focus on education, Dr. Roy became co-Principal Investigator on the FDA PDC grant and the engineering lead for the program. His leadership helped create a specific cadre of engineers, Master of Engineering students, and other interested industry engineers engaged and capable of participating in the innovation process.

As the Pediatric Device Consortium grew and both academic and commercial successes spun off from the enterprise, the Department of Surgery and UCSF Chancellors' Office both lent financial and personnel support to the program beyond pediatric devices. As such, the unique UCSF Pediatric Device Consortium expanded beyond pediatric devices to include adult devices and grew into UCSF Surgical Innovations. This established a formal program within the Department of Surgery, leading to resident training and more streamlined processes to initiate clinical testing. This has resulted in a consistent pipeline of talent, with additional support from a NIH-funded R25 grant for the Biodevice Innovation Training Program for surgical residents and the UC Berkeley-UCSF Master of Translational Medicine Program for budding engineers and device entrepreneurs. Within this ecosystem, Surgical Innovations has succeeded in nurturing the ideas of clinical faculty members in academia and creating the training structure and capacity to recruit surgical residents and engineers. This collaborative framework is reflected in Fig. 13.1.

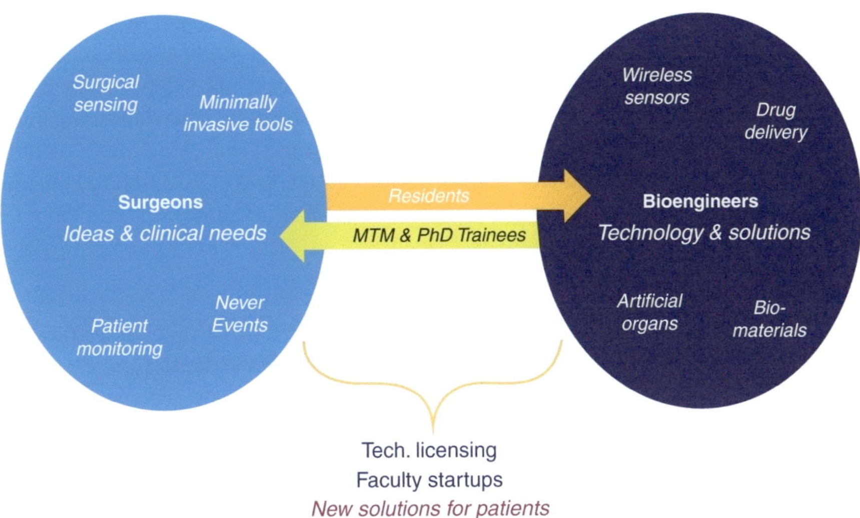

Fig. 13.1 Overview of the collaborative framework between clinicians and bioengineers

These collaborations and framework of talent and collaboration have led to significantly enhanced faculty inventions, involvement, and support. The total involvement to date includes 38 surgical faculty (greater than one-third of the department), 50 non-surgical faculty, over 50 bioengineering students, and eight trained surgical research fellows.

As an aggregate, the mission statement of UCSF Surgical Innovations is to accelerate the translation of pioneering medical devices to improve patient care by (1) Lowering the barriers for clinician-innovators by providing accessible infrastructure for device innovation, (2) Accelerating viable projects towards commercialization, and (3) Educating trainees in interdisciplinary collaboration and translation.

Partnerships with Industry to Create a Viable Ecosystem

Being based in the San Francisco Bay Area, there is a strong culture of innovation and entrepreneurship in the local business and startup ecosystem that permeates into the academic medical center. This has led to a push from the University of California, San Francisco, to develop one of their strategic goals, entitled the UCSF "Biosilicon Collaboratory," to develop high-impact external partnerships with industry and facilitate homegrown technological innovation. The early groundwork laid by the PDC and Surgical Innovations in creating new medical devices led to support from the UCSF Chancellor's Office, as it aligned with their strategic goal. This led to expansion of Surgical Innovations' reach beyond the scope of the Department of Surgery to all interventional departments. Since that time, we have successfully assisted projects in the fields of General Surgery, Cardiac Surgery, Vascular Surgery, Otolaryngology, Plastic Surgery, Neurosurgery, Orthopedic Surgery, Urology, Radiology, and Anesthesiology.

The Bay Area ecosystem also permitted us to tap into local resources and incubators, including partnerships with TheraNova, LLC. (a local medical device incubator), QB3 and the Rosenman Institute (a university-based life sciences incubator and entrepreneurship program), Zeus (an international medical materials company), Ansys (an engineering and design software company), and MedTech Venture Partners (a local medical technology venture capital firm). Additionally, many enthusiastic and experienced industry professionals have volunteered their time to serve as consultants for our initiatives.

Section 3: Building Capacity in Faculty and Resident Surgeons

While we have created a strong ecosystem for innovation and entrepreneurship in surgery, the foundational ideas and development come from faculty and resident surgeons themselves. This is a unique aspect of thinking in relation to surgical training. The foundation begins as an adjunct to longstanding meetings in an academic medical center setting. Biweekly hour-long meetings are held immediately after weekly Surgery Grand Rounds, with an additional Innovators Forum held one afternoon per week. These meetings function as a gathering for faculty and innovators to pitch their ideas to an interdisciplinary group of involved physicians, engineers, and individuals involved in medical device entrepreneurship. In addition, one of the Surgical Grand Rounds each quarter is a dedicated "Innovation Grand Rounds," serving as an opportunity for industry experts or advanced faculty in device development to present their innovations to the Department of Surgery as a whole.

Through these educational forums, naturally, collaborations are often formed. Whether due to similar interests or synergies from variable skill sets and domain expertise, these regular meetings provide a venue for like-minded surgeons and staff engineers to work together to think through solutions to clinical problems. To respect privacy and confidentiality, each meeting is protected by a "Code of Conduct" signed by all attendees external to the University of California system. This, then serving as a closed meeting, means that ideas presented are not considered public disclosures in relation to future patent filings, and there is a built-in protection component similar to a nondisclosure agreement (NDA). This further fosters a collaborative and safe environment to discuss new ideas, grow from mentorship, and receive constant feedback, iteration, and support from colleagues.

This collaborative environment has led to a scalable infrastructure capable of supporting many projects, expanding beyond the initial scope of the Department of Surgery. A total of 86 faculty members across 19 departments and schools are now involved in some capacity with UCSF Surgical Innovations, with the breakdown reflected in Fig. 13.2.

While both clinical and technical knowledge are needed to create a new device or technology, the long arc of development also requires a viable foundation for a future business, including a value proposition and the potential for market adoption. Our role in the process entails creating a framework combining medicine, engineering, and business through a two-pronged approach: securing funding and understanding the foundations of medical device entrepreneurship.

From a funding perspective, in addition to institutional and departmental funds, we assist faculty in applying for additional National Institutes of Health (NIH), National Science Foundation (NSF), and Small Business Innovation Research (SBIR) grants. From that point, through the "Biosilicon Collaboratory" network, additional introductions are made to possible investors, both in the scope of early-stage angel investors, and later stage venture capital firms and possible industry partners.

In regard to entrepreneurship, there is a broad scope of knowledge and industry expertise provided to the involved faculty, from educational seminars about general business principles to networking events. Our core competencies also include advising and hands-on guidance about understanding the regulatory (FDA) process, intellectual property considerations, licensing agreements and royalties, overcoming engineering challenges, establishing a development timeline, understanding the market positioning, creating a value proposition, navigating the competitive space,

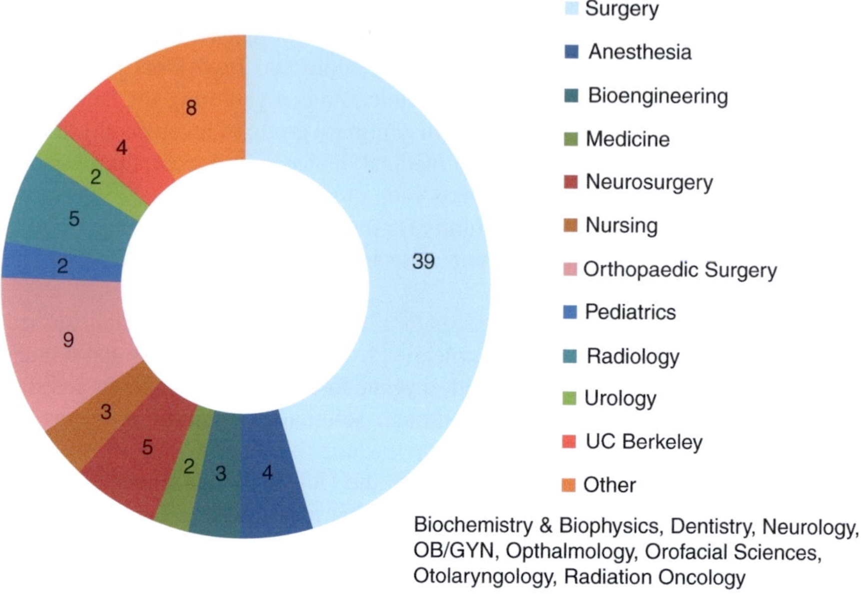

Fig. 13.2 Breakdown of projects by department

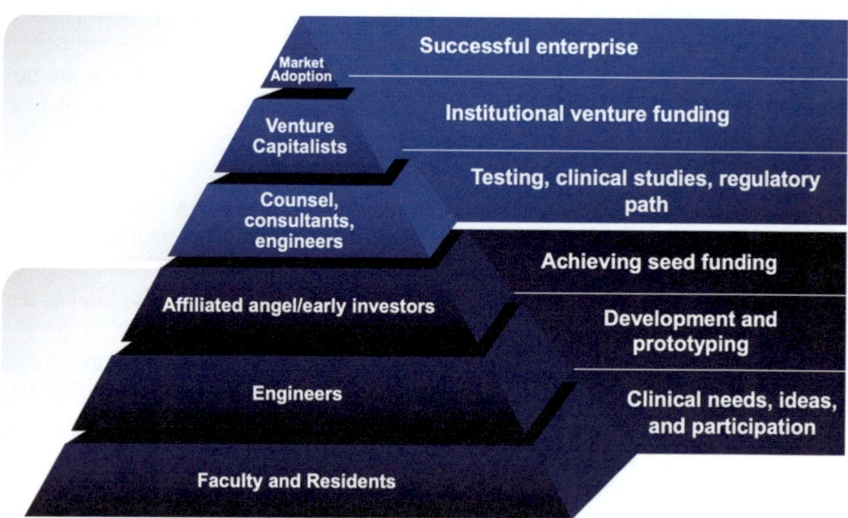

Fig. 13.3 Depiction of additional layers of capacity needed to achieve a successful enterprise

developing a commercialization plan, and understanding quality systems management for manufacturing. Figure 13.3 depicts our approach to building knowledge and providing support to faculty clinicians wishing to create a device or launch a new initiative.

Section 4: Stimulating Faculty Technology Development

While the initial impetus for the development of a clinical solution and project generally comes from one of the aforementioned brainstorming sessions or formal meetings, the roadmap to a successful endeavor reflects a long journey. Our institution has built a core infrastructure to take an idea from concept to prototype to testing. First, the process begins with assigning a team of interested engineers to a specific project based on their areas of expertise, with subsequent creation of goals and milestones jointly agreed upon with the engineers and the faculty physician. Second, we form a team of effective advisors around the concept, from entrepreneurs and business advisors to regulatory consultants and intellectual property counsel. This helps the project leader (traditionally a member of the surgical faculty) to create their own roadmap for success and gather advice and lead their team through further development of the project. The key is to not only build a successful prototype, but also combine novel engineering technologies, better define the clinical problem, and tailor a more effective solution with a viable future market position.

With the team intact and a roadmap for product development created, the next challenge for most enterprises still holds true here: funding. Funding, whether for entrepreneurial ventures or research projects, remains a key rate-limiting step, but essential component of future work. As such, most medical device companies falter during a phase known as the "Valley of Death." This is the point in the development cycle where there is not yet a sufficiently well validated concept or market appeal to create revenue generation or support outside investment, but the capital requirements to get to such a stage require more funds than the founders are capable of providing. The University of California, San Francisco, and the Department of Surgery have jointly created internal programs in order to bridge this critical gap. The University, through their Innovation Ventures fund, runs a program entitled the "UCSF Catalyst Program." This program provides up to $100,000 in seed funding for promising technologies across the University. Specifically, our division and the Department of Surgery have been remarkably successful in having many initiatives raise seed funding through this program, with the stipulation that early-stage intellectual property arising from the venture will be filed jointly with the University of California, and that the enterprise will have early access for future licensing of the technology.

Additionally, we have two internal pathways to smaller amounts of funding: one from the Department of Surgery and UCSF Chancellor's funds – creating the Surgical Innovations' Accelerator Program – and another from an FDA grant for the creation and maintenance of a Pediatric Device Consortium, specifically for pediatric initiatives.

As the projects become more sophisticated and move forward along their development pathway, the Surgical Innovations group strives to provide a multidisciplinary team for the surgeons. In addition to the engineers, advisors, and consultants mentioned above, a key part of the value from the center comes from the involvement and training of surgical residents. This has led to the creation of the

UCSF Biodevice Innovation Pathway, which has led to eight surgery residents who have thus far devoted their two research years to a formal education curriculum and hands-on experience and mentorship working on key projects. The fellowship consists of research, coursework, interdisciplinary meetings, mentorship, and experience in prototyping and development – with a goal towards practical learning and academic productivity to lay the foundation for future work in innovation in surgery.

Additional industry support is provided through collaboration agreements, with expertise in product development, regulatory affairs, intellectual property, entrepreneurship, guidance through a Commercialization Advisory Board, and any adjunct services accessible at any stage of the total product development lifecycle. Our group, in particular, specializes in guiding early stage endeavors from conception to prototype to proof-of-concept clinical testing, providing surgical faculty both the infrastructure and the wide breadth of resources needed.

Section 5: Overview of Successful Projects and Roadmap from Conception to Technology

Many successful projects have come through the UCSF Surgical Innovations program. Dr. Shuvo Roy has continued to advance his work in the creation of an artificial kidney and bioartificial pancreas. Dr. Shant Vartanian (Vascular Surgery) has developed a device for percutaneous AV Fistula creation, Dr. David Conrad (Otolaryngology) has created a wireless alarm to sense accidental decannulation of a tracheostomy tube, Dr. Matthew Haight and Dr. Merlin Larson (Anesthesiology) have developed a titratable method for epidural anesthesia, and Dr. Alexis Dang and Dr. Alex Dang (Orthopedic Surgery) have created a system to augment surgical vision and identification of tissue planes. Dr. Insoo Suh (Endocrine Surgery) has created the "Lamprey retractor" for atraumatic laparoscopic soft tissue manipulation and retraction, and Dr. Hanmin Lee (Pediatric Surgery) has led the "SmartDerm" project with a patch device and combined machine learning algorithms for real-time monitoring, prediction, and treatment of pressure ulcers. Additionally, Dr. Benjamin Padilla (Pediatric Surgery) has led a team in the creation of a High-Efficiency External Ambulatory Lung to develop a gas exchange membrane. Dr. Michael Harrison (Pediatric Surgery) has created Magnamosis for the creation of minimally invasive and safe bowel anastomoses, MagNap for the implantation of a magnet to the hyoid bone to create a new treatment of obstructive sleep apnea, an implantable magnetic device for the correction of pectus excavatum, and an expandable implanted rod for orthopedic surgery and correction of scoliosis. Dr. Matthew Lin (Minimally Invasive Surgery) has created an articulating endoscopic grasper, and Dr. Georg Wieselthaler (Cardiac Surgery) has developed an implantable sensor that can monitor for graft rejection after cardiac transplantation. These are just a selection of the many projects in the Surgical Innovations group, and reflect the impact of combining the collective clinical knowledge of surgical faculty with the support of a dedicated team of residents and engineers in conjunction with the infrastructure needed to drive these initiatives forward.

The majority of these technologies and ideas came from a clinician expressing a clinical need and presenting at one of the weekly Innovators Forums, which includes attendees comprised of clinicians, engineers, trainees, and industry professionals. The discussion is guided by comprehensive consideration of the clinical merits, technical nuances, market evaluation, value proposition, regulatory path, intellectual property, and commercialization potential. Thereafter, a team of engineers, either in-house talent, or a Masters in Engineering team, is assigned to the project and guided by the faculty physician.

To date, eight projects are currently in human clinical trials, and another nine are in animal studies. In total, nine faculty startups have been created and spun off from the Surgical Innovations program and over $30 million has been raised from outside sources for future work.

Section 6: Future Directions

Our experiences provide one roadmap for creating a multidisciplinary surgical innovations group at an academic medical center and stimulating surgery faculty technology development. What began has an informal meeting of like-minded and innovative surgeons has blossomed over a decade into a much larger initiative. However, many of the original tenets and lessons learned from earlier successful technological innovation continue to hold true – it takes a group of motivated individuals from diverse backgrounds working towards a common goal, with support, mentorship, and feedback guiding daily advances. Surgeons are involved early as creative partners with engineers, and their joint expertise results in combining clinical need and new technologies to create viable solutions. One of the greatest lessons learned includes the need to foster and maintain a culture of innovation and respect across disciplines – one where new ideas are accepted and critical feedback discussed, with a common goal to bring forth new solutions for our patients.

One of the continuing challenges remaining is one seen across many industries and enterprises – the need for scalable solutions and ongoing growth. As one device succeeds, we find that the lessons learned help guide others, and bring forth additional support from industry and investors in both the local and national ecosystem. We are learning that such an ecosystem warrants a continuum of support for innovation all along an idea's path, from realization to a scalable and viable solution. Therefore, we are working to integrate what are currently discrete entities of support (need-finding, early stage prototyping, fundraising, etc.) at each stage of the product's development, and create better "handoff" points from one group to the next.

We believe that we are uniquely suited to address these challenges through our ability to soften departmental boundaries using a shared institutional mission. Looking towards the future, we also believe that one of the most important reasons for the program's continued success will be a diverse, multi-faceted support system with representatives from industry, investment, and academic communities. Going forward, we are looking to continue strengthening both of these support systems to enable a single, seamless pipeline of innovation with the continued mission to decrease the barriers to innovation for clinicians, accelerate viable projects towards commercialization, and educate trainees to lead innovation in medicine – all for one common goal: to improve care for our patients.

Chapter 14
Engaging SBIR Resources for Development of Surgical Innovations in Oncology

Deepa Narayanan, Christie A. Canaria, Monique Pond, and Michael Weingarten

Introduction

The overarching goal of this chapter is to demonstrate how the National Cancer Institute (NCI)'s Small Business Innovation Research (SBIR)/Small Business Technology Transfer (STTR) program can be leveraged to foster, develop, and translate surgical technologies into the commercial space so that investigators, innovators, and entrepreneurs will utilize the products to enhance health, lengthen life, and reduce illness and disability. Through a combination of funding and non-funding resources, NCI SBIR is committed to supporting early stage technology development, including those arising from research institutions and academia, towards the commercial space where they can be accessed by and serve patients.

Overview of the SBIR/STTR Program

The SBIR program was established by the United States (U.S.) Congress in 1982 to strengthen the role of innovative small business concerns (SBCs) in federally-funded research or research and development (R&D). It requires federal agencies with extramural R&D budgets that exceed $100 million to set aside 3.2% to fund small business awards. In 1992, the STTR program was established and requires agencies with extramural R&D budgets exceeding $1 billion to set aside an additional 0.45% to support STTR awards for small businesses. The major

D. Narayanan (✉) · C. A. Canaria · M. Pond · M. Weingarten
National Cancer Institute, Rockville, MD, USA
e-mail: deepa.narayanan@nih.gov; christie.canaria@nih.gov; monique.pond@nih.gov; weingartenm@mail.nih.gov

© Springer Nature Switzerland AG (outside the USA) 2019
M. S. Cohen, L. Kao (eds.), *Success in Academic Surgery: Innovation and Entrepreneurship*, Success in Academic Surgery,
https://doi.org/10.1007/978-3-030-18613-5_14

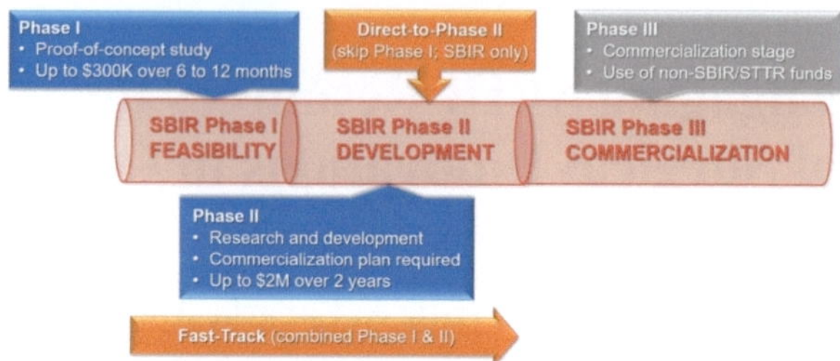

Fig. 14.1 Three phases of funding for Federal SBIR and STTR programs

distinguishing feature of the STTR program is that projects must involve a cooperative R&D arrangement between small businesses and research institutions. In 2018, NIH's SBIR/STTR programs invested over $1 billion into health and life science companies that are creating innovative technologies that align with NIH's mission to improve health and save lives. To be eligible to apply for SBIR or STTR awards, the SBC must be a for-profit, U.S.-owned small business with fewer than 500 employees. Eligibility requirements for the SBIR/STTR program are defined by Small Business Administration Regulations at 13 C.F.R. § 121.701–705 [1]. The funding structure of the NCI SBIR/STTR programs is composed of three phases, which are described in Fig. 14.1. Traditionally, resources are competed as a Phase I award followed by Phase II award. The Fast-Track option allows companies to apply for Phase I and Phase II funding simultaneously to decrease the time between individual awards. The Direct-to-Phase II option, exclusively offered for the SBIR program, allows companies without a prior Phase I award to apply directly for Phase II funding support if they have completed the equivalent of Phase I work previously.

NCI SBIR Development Center

Among the 27 NIH institutes, the National Cancer Institute (NCI) has the largest SBIR/STTR program with an annual budget of $167 million; these programs serve as the primary NCI resource for supporting the development, translation, and ultimate commercialization of high-impact, biomedical technologies that prevent, diagnose, and treat cancer-related diseases. Based on the recent *1998-2018 National Economic Impacts* report from the National Cancer Institute SBIR/STTR Program, NCI invested ***$787 million in to small businesses through 690 separate Phase II awards,which resulted in*** $26.1 billion in total economic output nationwide [2]. That's a 33:1 return on the NCI's investment and a testament to the value and impact of the SBIR/STTR program. The NCI Development Center (the "Center") has a centralized model for managing SBIR/STTR programs with a full staff that oversee both technical and commercialization aspects of awards. The main function of the Center is to provide central oversight to a portfolio of over 400 active projects and to seed emerging technology areas by developing targeted funding opportunities either as grants or contracts. In addition, Center staff is responsible for advising applicants about potential funding options and providing application tips [2]. The Center conducts over 30 outreach events each year in cities across the U.S. to attract quality applicants and raise awareness of the program on a national level. Another important goal of the Center is to facilitate connections between NCI SBIR portfolio companies and potential investors/strategic partners to continue development of technology post SBIR funding. The Center also provides training to applicants in the form of non-funding assistance programs such as entrepreneurial training programs, workshops, and webinars, which will be discussed in detail in the subsequent pages.

Surgical Innovations Portfolio

Information about all NIH and NCI funded projects is publicly available using the NIH Reporter Database (https://projectreporter.nih.gov/reporter.cfm). Using keywords such as "surgery", "surgical tools", "margins", "NIR", "interventional", and "intraoperative", this database was mined to identify surgical technologies funded by NCI SBIR in the past 10 years. The list of awards was manually curated to remove technologies that were oncology drugs, diagnostic imaging, or in vitro diagnostic technologies. NCI SBIR has funded 127 surgical technologies between fiscal years 2009 and 2018 (Fig. 14.2), including 70 Phase I awards to study feasibility and 57 Phase II awards for advanced R&D to expand and develop the Phase I

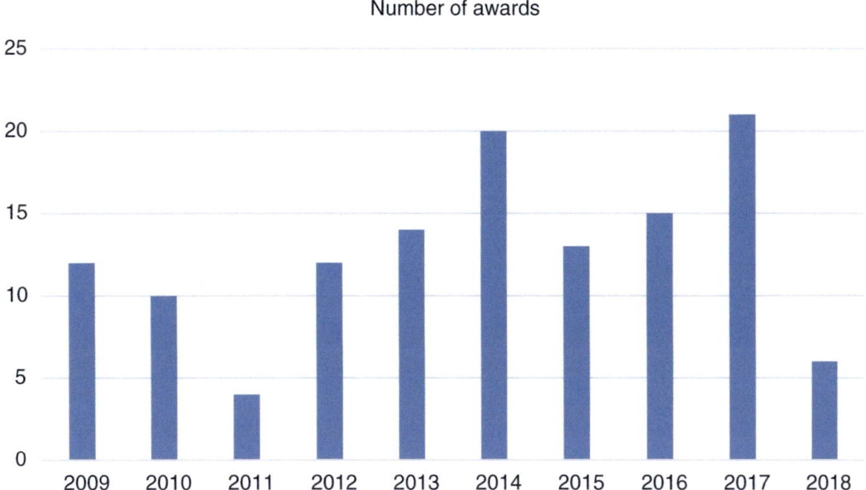

Fig. 14.2 Number of surgical technologies funded by the NCI SBIR Development Center from 2009 to 2018

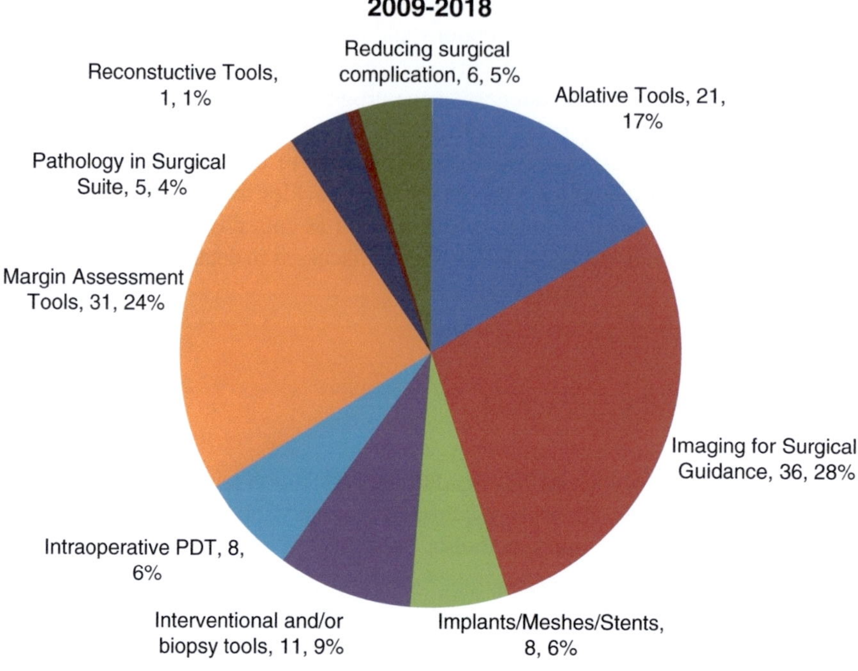

Fig. 14.3 Types of technologies funded by the NCI SBIR Development Center

concept. A breakdown of the types of technologies funded by SBIR is shown in Fig. 14.3. One active area for start-ups in the surgical space is the development of imaging tools to optimize surgical guidance including Magnetic Resonance Imaging (MRI), optical imaging, Computerized Tomography (CT) imaging, Positron Emission Mammography (PET) Imaging, Optical Coherence Tomography, Near Infrared Imaging, and Ultrasound imaging technologies along with image processing and image registration tools. Additional active areas of research are tools and technologies for margin assessment in cancer resection for all types of cancers including breast, cervical, ovarian, melanoma, lung, colorectal, and prostate cancers.

Innovative surgical tools often require considerable financing beyond the SBIR Phase II award to complete the necessary validation studies and/or clinical trials for regulatory approval. In addition to the Phase I and Phase II funding, the NCI Phase IIB Bridge Award Program helps promising SBCs address the funding gap between the end of the SBIR Phase II award and commercialization, commonly known as the "Valley of Death". Companies that are developing cancer-related technologies with a Phase II SBIR or STTR award from any federal agency are eligible to apply for the Phase IIB Bridge Award of up to $4 million. The Phase IIB Bridge Award incentivizes partnerships between successful Phase II small businesses and private investors by providing competitive preference to applicants that can secure non-federal matching funds (1:1 minimum) during the Bridge Award project period. One of the companies to receive a Phase IIB Bridge Award was Fibralign Corporation (Union City CA, https://www.fibralignbio.com) for prospective evaluation of a surgical solution for breast cancer associated lymphedema. Prior to receiving NCI support, Fibralign utilized SBIR Phase I and II funding from the Department of Defense and National Science Foundation (NSF) to develop its Nanoweave nanofibrillar scaffolds in aid of lymphatic tissue regeneration. Building on that technology, Fibralign is now developing BioBridge as a novel, thread-like collagen scaffold designed to support the regeneration of new healthy lymphatic vessels that will repair diseased tissue in patients that are suffering from breast cancer-related lymphedema. Using the NCI SBIR funds, they plan to evaluate the efficacy of BioBridge in 75 patients that have Stage II or Stage III breast cancer-related lymphedema in a multi-site clinical study led by Stanford University.

Non-Funding Resources

The SBIR/STTR programs provide small businesses with valuable funding to complete the pre-clinical and prototyping studies needed to translate promising technologies into prospective clinical trials. While funding is important, other resources are similarly critical. The Center currently provides a range of training opportunities and resources to assist current SBIR/STTR applicants and awardees including program staff guidance, workshops and webinars, entrepreneurship training, and investor engagement (Fig. 14.4). Feedback on these programs has been overwhelmingly positive, and participating companies have achieved many positive outcomes and significant commercialization milestones. Experience with these initiatives suggests that mentoring assistance, development and commercialization training, and networking with business experts can substantially affect the success of translating research projects to the clinic.

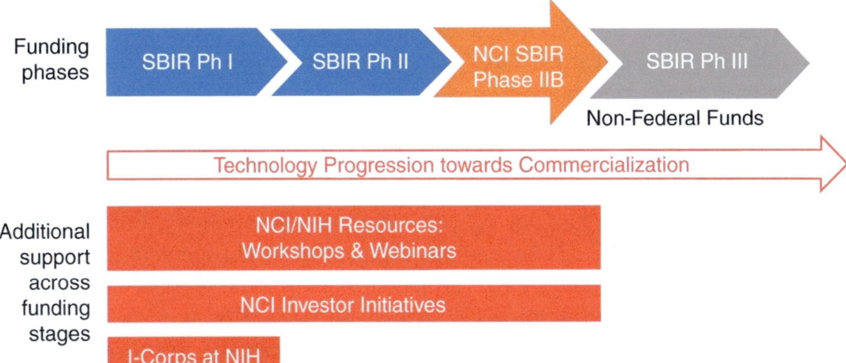

Fig. 14.4 NCI SBIR Development Center Resources for Small Businesses

The Center is staffed with program directors possessing broad technology expertise and experience in small business R&D, federal regulatory pathway, and technology commercialization strategy. Program directors are available to engage with potential applicants prior to submitting proposals; investigators, even those that have not yet established a small business, are encouraged to engage with staff before they apply. Across the country in person and virtually, program staff connect with pre-applicants to review the SBIR programs and discuss alignment of technology applications with the NCI mission. With three standard submission dates scheduled annually (January 5, April 5, and September 5), investigators can connect with program staff throughout the year, as schedules allow. For logistics purposes, NCI SBIR encourages applicants to contact staff at least a month before the intended submission deadline.

SBIR/STTR Phase I awardees are eligible to compete for supplemental resources including the Innovation Corps (I-Corps™ at NIH) program, an 8-week immersive training program that teaches researchers and technologists how to apply the scientific method to the entrepreneurship process (https://www.sbir.cancer.gov/icorps). Through I-Corps at NIH, small businesses receive entrepreneurial training to create a business model and explore the technology ecosystem surrounding their potential product. I-Corps emphasizes participant engagement and getting out of the building to talk to key stakeholders and potential customers to inform the business model. The Center manages the I-Corps program, which includes 22 NIH Institutes/Centers and the Centers for Disease Control and Prevention (CDC). Since the launch of the program in 2014, more than 140 teams with projects ranging from therapeutics to surgical devices have explored the entrepreneurial landscape to identify a path for technology commercialization.

One such participant, IGI Technologies, Inc. (College Park, MD), is developing an augmented reality solution for laparoscopic surgery. The medical device fuses live ultrasound images with traditional laparoscopic images to guide surgeons in performing minimally invasive procedures faster and with more confidence. Prior to embarking on the I-Corps program in 2014, IGI Technologies had spoken with clinicians at their partner institute to identify usability pain points in ultrasound imaging for clinicians employing laparoscopy techniques. IGI Technologies came into I-Corps thinking that surgeons would leap at the opportunity to use their augmented reality technology, but learned through key interviews with stakeholders that the rate of laparoscopic surgery *with ultrasound* was significantly lower than initially hypothesized. By getting out of the building and talking to people outside their immediate community, the company identified and validated several surgical subspecialties as users for the technology, like surgical oncology and urology, and also a new sub-specialty they had not yet considered: thoracic surgery. Based on their learnings during I-Corps, IGI Technologies expanded its engagement to address a wider surgical market and formed partnerships with adult surgical centers. IGI Technologies continues to develop its device with support from a Phase II STTR grant; the team has also taken advantage of NCI programming and NCI organized workshops.

The Development Center offers small business applicants and awardees educational opportunities including the Peer Learning and Networking (PLAN) webinar series and workshops to provide resources to expedite commercialization. As part of the PLAN webinar series, funded companies share their specific expertise with their peer awardees. The webinar series aims to incentivize peer learning and provide small businesses with networking opportunities. NCI also organizes biennial workshops (TRECS), providing NCI awardees an opportunity to learn about federal and non-federal resources that are available for advancing commercialization and supporting opportunities for networking with other awardees. At the last workshop held in May 2018, panels featured representatives from the Food and Drug Administration (FDA), Center for Medicaid and Medicare Services (CMS), Congressionally Directed Medical Research Programs (CDMRP), NSF, and other NCI specific resource programs. The expert panelists also participated in one-on-one meetings with attendees and provided them the opportunity to receive in-depth suggestions or guidance that could propel the company's commercialization efforts. The 2018 NCI SBIR TRECS Workshop ended with positive feedback from attendees, with 96% of surveyed attendees finding the workshop mostly to entirely valuable.

Developing tools from the lab to the clinic typically requires external funding in addition to federal funding. The NCI SBIR program understands that facilitating connections between small businesses and potential investors is essential to get technologies to the clinic. The Center's Investor Initiatives program provides an opportunity for promising NCI-funded small businesses to showcase their technologies to investors and strategic partners. The SBIR program recruits a panel of 50–60 external reviewers with industry and venture backgrounds to review applications and selects about 25–30 companies to present at various events such as MedTech Innovator, Life Science Summit, BioNetwork, and Personalized Medicine World Conference. The program provides pitch coaching, support to present at an industry event, and the potential for one-on-one meetings with investors and strategic partners.

In the past 10 years, surgical innovation tools have made up 9.2% (127/1385) of the NCI SBIR grant portfolio. Several companies have successfully leveraged SBIR funding and resources to translate technologies from academia into the clinic. One such company is OnTarget Laboratories (West Lafayette, IN, www.ontargetlaboratories.com), which is developing a cancer-targeted fluorescent marker to aid surgeons in tumor resection. OnTarget Laboratories (OTL) was originally founded in 2010 based on work in Prof. Philip Low's lab at Purdue University. The innovation began when then-graduate student Sumith Kularatne (now Executive VP of R&D) and Low were able to demonstrate selective uptake of tumor-targeted drugs to cancer cells. The technology was spun out into OTL as an intraoperative research tool to assist surgeons in identifying and resecting tumor tissue. Since then, the Indiana-based company has been developing agents to address a number of solid tumors. For many hi-tech small business endeavors, the earliest support is sourced from friends and family, as was true for OTL; co-founders Philip Low and Martin Low (CEO) are brothers and serial entrepreneurs. However, there exists a broader ecosystem of support for small businesses to move their technologies forward. Among the resources are federal SBIR/

STTR funding, state funding, more traditional venture capital, and strategic partnerships, each of which can be integral in supporting small businesses during R&D intensive times. In 2015, OTL received NCI SBIR Phase I funding to support feasibility studies for its lead compound in intra-operative use during lung cancer resection. In 2016, OTL participated in NCI SBIR Investor Initiatives and received support from NCI to attend a technology showcase event with JLABS Boston. In 2017, OTL received SBIR Phase II funding to support additional R&D activity. That same year, through diligence discussions that were helped by their presentation at the NCI SBIR Investor Initiatives event, OTL secured $32.5 million in financing from Johnson and Johnson Innovation. Soon thereafter, the company captured an additional $11.1 million in financing led by H.I.G. BioHealth Partners, Elevate Ventures and Helsinn to close their Series B round. Today, this technology, which started at the university bench, has evolved into the company lead target (OTL38) and is in Phase 3 clinical trials for ovarian cancer and Phase 2 clinical trials for lung cancer inflammatory disease. Surgeons both domestically and internationally are using OTL's technology during cancer resection surgeries and attest to its power in improving outcomes in surgery and for patients. With OTL tools, surgeons can remove 5× more cancer with the aid of fluorescent markers than without it [3]. That's a key value proposition for a technology in the surgical suite because a successful surgery that removes all of the tumor can significantly increase overall patient survival.

In addition to these NCI specific programs, companies can take advantage of assistance programs conducted by the NIH. The NIH manages two program opportunities each year that provide technical assistance to small business awardees including the Niche Assessment Program (NAP) and the Commercialization Accelerator Program (CAP). The NAP program aims to jump-start commercialization efforts by providing Phase I awardees with market analysis assistance. The CAP is a 9-month individualized assistance program for Phase II awardees. Both programs have a competitive application process but are complimentary to participants. As the innovation climate changes, NCI and NIH are constantly piloting new funding and assistance programs.

Spurring Academic Innovations

Innovation does not exist in a vacuum. The ecosystem supporting technology development is made up of multiple stakeholders. Small businesses assume great risk in developing early-stage technologies, and public funding resources exist at the federal and state levels. Private and strategic partnerships provide additional assistance, and often, research institutions help create and collaborate on many of these innovative ideas.

Academic investigators make significant contributions to NCI-funded SBIR and STTR projects–24/127 projects in the surgical technology space were STTR grants.

STTR grants require higher involvement from research institutions, (e.g. universities); at least 30% of the work must be done at the institution, and it allows for greater flexibility for the Principal Investigator to retain an academic affiliation and still be part of the small business. A recent portfolio analysis of FY 2017 NCI awards revealed that $18 million (17%) of SBIR and $9 million (44%) of STTR grant funding was subcontracted to academic institutions. While these data indicate that academic investigators routinely participate in the SBIR/STTR programs, new strategies to better assist academics may accelerate commercialization of innovations discovered in university laboratories.

Indeed, universities house a rich pool of basic science projects on which translational technology is built. Within the U.S., such institutions vary in size, location, programmatic focus, and approach to translational science. In short, there is great diversity across establishment cultures. Since the creation of the SBIR and STTR programs, there has been a shift in attitudes and the roles of universities in developing innovative technologies. For example, Dartmouth College in New Hampshire serves approximately 6500 students (undergraduate and graduate combined) and has more than 50 research-focused centers, institutes, and groups in areas ranging from 'medicine and the arts' to 'engineering and business'. Dartmouth has embraced a progressive approach to technology development and reduced barriers across traditionally siloed schools such as business and engineering. One such return on Dartmouth's innovation investment is CairnSurgical, Inc. (Lebanon, NH), a collaborative effort co-founded with researchers across the campus: Richard Barth, MD is Professor of Surgery at Geisel School of Medicine; Keith Paulsen, PhD is Professor of Biomedical Engineering and Scientific Director of the Center for Surgical Innovation at Dartmouth-Hitchcock Medical Center; and Venkat Krishnaswamy, PhD is former Assistant Professor from the Thayer School of Engineering.

CairnSurgical is a clinical stage company developing the Breast Cancer Locator (BCL) system for use in breast lumpectomy procedures. BCL supports surgeons in localizing and resecting palpable and non-palpable tumors in order to improve both procedure outcomes and costs [4]. CairnSurgical has received SBIR funding in the form of Phase I, Phase II, and Fast-Track grants. Prior to securing federal resources, the investigators benefitted from the support of their local ecosystem. In 2014, Barth received the Dartmouth SYNERGY Clinician-Entrepreneur Fellowship, a program designed to develop entrepreneurial skills among Dartmouth clinical faculty for the commercialization of innovations and inventions that address patient care needs. In 2017, CairnSurgical also received New Hampshire state grant funding to support technology innovation in collaboration with academia. In 2018, CairnSurgical leveraged these resources to secure additional programmatic support from the NCI Investor Initiatives program to attend the 2018 Med Alley Innovation Summit. CairnSurgical is an example of a small business taking advantage of the ecosystem and the breadth of the ecosystem, among which the SBIR/STTR program sits.

Summary

Surgical technologies represent a critical part of the NCI SBIR portfolio, and the NCI SBIR program has supported the development of a number of new surgical tools aimed at alleviating the burden of cancer. Both funding and non-funding resources are essential for commercialization and clinical adoption of novel cancer technologies. Understanding challenges and early predictors of success in the development of surgical tools is critical to identify the optimal funding and non-funding resources to support start-ups in this space. NCI SBIR is focused on improving the SBIR program and continues to engage in outreach to raise awareness of the program and reach underserved populations and geographic areas to attract quality applicants developing innovative technologies. Start-ups seeking funding to commercialize promising surgical tools and technologies are encouraged to contact a NCI SBIR program director to discuss their projects. Center staff are available to assist with providing guidance regarding resources to speed the clinical adoption of surgical innovations. By empowering entrepreneurs at small businesses, NCI SBIR aims to increase the translation of innovative cancer-related research into commercialized technologies available for clinicians, patients, and their families in support of NIH's mission to help all people live longer, healthier lives.

References

1. https://www.govinfo.gov.
2. Deepa Narayanan, Michael Weingarten, Chapter 9 - An Introduction to the National Institutes of Health SBIR/STTR Programs, Editor(s): Kevin E. Behrns, Bruce Gingles, Michael G. Sarr, Medical Innovation, Academic Press, 2018, Pages 87-100, ISBN 9780128149263, https://sbir.cancer.gov/sites/default/files/documents/NCI_SBIR_ImpactStudy_FullReport.pdf Accessed May 6, 2019
3. van Dam GM, Themelis G, Crane LM, Harlaar NJ, Pleijhuis RG, Kelder W, Sarantopoulos A, de Jong JS, Arts HJ, van der Zee AG, Bart J, Low PS, Ntziachristos V. Intraoperative tumor-specific fluorescence imaging in ovarian cancer by folate receptor-α targeting: first in-human results. Nat Med. 2011;17:1315–9.
4. Barth RJ, Krishnaswamy V, Paulsen KD, et al. A patient-specific 3D-printed form accurately transfers supine MRI-derived tumor localization information to guide breast-conserving surgery. Ann Surg Oncol. 2017;24:2950–6.

Chapter 15
Creating ROI: Return on Innovation-the Partners Model

Ronald G. Tompkins, Andrew K. Alexander, and Carl M. Berke

New Technology Must Be Translated into Products to Benefit Patients

Healthcare Customers Expect Innovation to Improve Care and Cost-Effectiveness

Multiple complex challenges create an increasing demand for better and more cost-effective healthcare solutions. Many healthcare markets increasingly include aging populations with multiple chronic diseases, cancer, and obesity to name a few very expensive challenges. US healthcare system expenditures for chronic disease management annually exceed $1 T and for management of diabetes, heart failure, and chronic obstructive pulmonary (COPD) alone, costs are $367B [1]. Furthermore, healthcare inflation, increasing regulatory requirements, higher liability for patient safety, and an evolving NIH emphasis of basic over translational science all provide additional barriers to innovation by academic medical centers (AMCs) and their interactions with industry. Ironically however, at the same time, AMCs are expected to lead in the innovation process by addressing all of these modern challenges in healthcare.

In fact, the public expects AMCs to lead in innovation partly because of their dominant and critical role in US healthcare delivery and partly because they rely

R. G. Tompkins (✉) · A. K. Alexander
Department of Surgery, Massachusetts General Hospital, Harvard Medical School, Boston, MA, USA
e-mail: rtompkins@mgh.harvard.edu; aalexander3@mgh.harvard.edu

C. M. Berke
Partners Healthcare Innovation, Partner, Partners Innovation Fund, Cambridge, MA, USA
e-mail: cberke@partners.org

© Springer Nature Switzerland AG 2019

205

M. S. Cohen, L. Kao (eds.), *Success in Academic Surgery: Innovation and Entrepreneurship*, Success in Academic Surgery,
https://doi.org/10.1007/978-3-030-18613-5_15

heavily on public funding intended to enable discovery in the biomedical sciences. In 1980, the Bayh-Dole Act granted title to intellectual property (IP) generated by inventions funded by the federal government to universities, small businesses, and nonprofit organizations, which further solidified the role of AMCs in biomedical science and healthcare innovation [2]. Academic institutions that emphasize innovation as important in their mission have made efforts to promote entrepreneurial cultures in their investigator communities, which collaborate with startup, pharmaceutical, and medical device companies to translate their academic inventions into commercial products for the benefit of society.

The relationship between AMCs and industry has resulted in increasingly defined but evolving professional and institutional conflict of interest policies. These policies are intended to protect against perceptions and realities of potential harms and abuse derived from financial incentives held by inventors and their academic institutions [3, 4]. Previous policies had been designed to avoid conflict by simply prohibiting these interactions [5, 6]. Increasingly, these evolving policies are being designed to recognize the benefits of public-private collaboration and to permit opportunities for these interactions while still maintaining patient safety and actively managing to minimize risk of bias and abuse introduced by these financial incentives.

Professional and institutional conflict policies have been crafted to accomplish a balance between the support of the innovative process and protections from any potential or actual harm. Previously, the balance had been tilted, without restraint, toward risk aversion by the institution prohibiting any support for innovation from healthcare industry suppliers who listen to voice of the customer in the market.

Currently many AMCs have taken critical steps to evolve their critical role to promote this translational process - one example has been the adoption of a "rebuttable presumption" approach. Although the institutional policies set conservative presumptions for faculty behavior regarding potential conflicts, administrative processes are beginning to review applications to better understand any potential conflicts and to allow the faculty to rebut these presumptions on a case-by-case basis. These applications request a waiver of one or more aspects of the presumption (i.e. rebuttal of the presumptions). If the faculty's rebuttal argument is convincing, a waiver may be allowed. In these cases, institutional management plans are typically initiated to monitor any real or potential conflicts by the faculty member in their developing relationship with industry or further development of their inventions.

Discovery and Invention Are Not Innovation Until They Reach the Market

Before embarking on innovation, a deep understanding of the unmet need is critical for ultimate success. From the innovator's perspective, the customer voice requires considerable work to clearly identify the problem that is being solved and to understand how each constituency in the healthcare system perceives the problem.

A clinician may be the end user of the product, but the purchase decision is made by the provider institution and they will be sensitive to the payer's willingness to reimburse. Clinicians are also not monolithic in their interpretation of an innovation's merit. It is a challenge to define a single solution to simultaneously meet all relative customer's needs. For example, in the field of bone marrow transplantation, even for cancer, there is little agreement among oncologists that the transplanted bone marrow cells should be purified to be cancer-free although this might be considered by some to be an obvious requirement.

Once a need is identified, which addresses a sufficiently large market that would justify the commitment of resources, it will be necessary to ensure that the technological challenges are understood well enough to be confident that these challenges can be overcome within a timeframe that is realistic. Ideally, technical challenges can be mitigated using institutional funding, perhaps even using federal funds, as a preamble to company creation. The more that the risk of the commercial proposition can be reduced prior to approaching potential investors, the easier it becomes to raise capital to create a venture for product development.

If the invention addresses a well-defined need that is significant enough to be worth solving and the technological risks are sufficiently understood and overcome, then investors can make a judgment as to whether, just because one can, a product development program should be pursued based on the invention, (i.e. Will the effort be worth it?). It is best to "fail fast" before too much effort and money has been spent for naught. An inventor or inventors who are so focused as to not be willing to walk away when confronted with reality could become a red flag to institutions and any potential investors. Frequently, the ultimate successful products from startup companies have not been the company's initial concepts but are altered versions that may not even resemble those concepts from the starting point.

There are many barriers to success in the market even if sufficient, initial financial investment has been garnered. Often timing is an important consideration – if a target innovation is too far ahead of customer awareness of the needs being addressed, adoption will be exceedingly delayed and revenue will be exhausted as subsequent investors lose patience. The challenge then becomes to prepare the market by educating customers to their value proposition. This is particularly challenging if the innovation is not a direct substitute with extra benefits for a product the customer is already using. The best combination is for the innovation to be an obvious improvement that customers would immediately understand and promptly switch to adopt. This requires careful planning and selection of the invention from the very beginning to ensure it will meet the needs of the market when it launches years after it was initiated.

Consider an example from our experience: a lab-on-a-chip diagnostic test for staging HIV disease in low-resource field settings. The technology was designed to determine if a patient's current therapy is working based upon thresholds for CD4 T-cell count. These T-cell counts would guide the decision to change treatments at the point of care. Over the multi-year course of the product development process, the market shifted to quantitative viral load rather than T-cell counts, making the innovative technology for a hematologic analysis no longer relevant despite the elegance of the solution.

On the other hand, the timing can be late by introducing a product whose value proposition is minimally better than the current product, which addresses the same or very similar need. In this case, the startup company product is competing on terms other than its exclusivity to adequately address a need. This problem becomes compounded when the competing product is marketed by a large, well established company with a tremendous advertising and marketing budget, sales force, and established customer base. The option for the startup is to compete based upon price, which means the startup must maintain a very low cost of goods, inventory, distribution, and customer support. Because of this very minor advantage to its value proposition, the startup's product becomes a commodity. Typically, venture investors shy away from investment in products that will become commodities because of their highly restricted return on investment, particularly when compared to the return on investment for a therapeutic.

An ideal innovation solves the well-defined need using well-understood technology (i.e. no eureka moment required) before formation of the company. Even after these conditions are met, there are multiple business challenges that remain, providing significant risk for a successful execution of the company. These include: regulatory, marketing, sales, competition, supply, distribution, manufacturing, and market adoption, to name a few, and any of these can contribute risk to ultimate business success. Invention can only be accepted as an innovation after it experiences an ultimately successful introduction of the product into the market.

Only Companies Can Supply Products, Not Hospitals or Professional Practices

Companies are in the business to compete and commercialize products by achieving the rights to sell products, to create barriers for others to sell the same or comparable products based upon regulatory approval, to organize the marketing and sales force identifying customers for these sales, to enable and ensure that these products are sold and reimbursed, to maintain an inventory of products, and to provide long term customer support among many other company activities. The company maintains and supports the product sales and distributions either directly or by using original equipment manufacturers (OEMs), distributors, or other vendors. Hospitals and professional practices can develop and support protocols and practice guidelines but in general, they do not routinely replace the many company activities for a successful innovation; those activities are most appropriately handled by a commercial entity.

The biomedical industry has evolved to a point where pharma and medtech practice an "open innovation" model in which companies seek out invention from academic wellsprings of discovery. Suppliers and manufacturers can fill their development pipelines by in-sourcing early stage programs from researchers and their host institutions who offer new and novel biological and clinical insights. This should be viewed as a healthy "ecology" in which the cooperating parties bring complementary expertise and resources to bear on important problems of commercial relevance ultimately for the benefit of public health.

Clinicians-Scientists Are Well Positioned to Find Solutions to Unmet Needs

Clinicians and scientists in academic medical centers routinely see clinical problems whose current solutions fall short of satisfaction by either the patient or the practitioner. Often, they are also in a position to ask "why" do we treat these conditions in this manner and "could there be better solutions" based on more recent scientific or technology advances? This creates a fertile environment for potential invention leading to innovation. There is a competitive advantage to the AMC setting that derives from the juxtaposition of practitioners of clinical medicine, basic science, engineering, and technology, who can provide solutions, with the clinicians, who are on the front lines of patient care (Fig. 15.2). The required clinical and technological interaction is promoted by the co-location of laboratory and clinic where collaborations can be initiated by encounters in a seminar, a grand rounds presentation, or in the cafeteria [7]. As is often the case, the training embodied in an MD/PhD graduate can converge the problem-solution capability in multiple of these domains within the same individual.

The benefits of clinician-scientist interaction can occur within an AMC's own investigator community, but it is equally productive when it happens through industry-academic cooperation. These creative encounters are promoted through conference participation, sponsored research agreements, industry-funded grant programs, crossover hiring, journal publication, and patent application filings to name a few examples.

Limitations of Traditional Tech Transfer Model

Bridging the Development Chasm Between Invention and Innovation

By far, the risk of failure because of the chasm between invention and actual achievement of innovation (e.g. commercialization) can be reduced by the many features mentioned above including: a greater understanding of the actual market need, the technology challenges, the clinical problem, the regulatory barriers, the scale-up challenges, the competitive landscape, the payment or reimbursement challenges, and a multitude of other more complex features related to successful development of a business startup (Fig. 15.1). This is just to mention a few of the challenges that create chaos and result in failures of what otherwise might be rational innovation in healthcare and medicine. One approach to reduce these risks is to remain in an incubation mode within an AMC while understanding and defining each of these risks and developing management strategies to mitigate them. This approach is easier to accomplish for devices and diagnostics rather than therapeutics. In this continuum, there is an advantage to begin with the clinical problem and to then explore technological options to create a meaningful solution within the AMC environment before venturing out into a startup company.

Although this can be a rational approach to increase the likelihood of success to cross this chasm, funding and managing the many challenges for academic incubation is also daunting. Over the past decade or more, there has been an increasing appreciation for a mutual interest shared between entrepreneurial young surgical scientists and their respective AMCs and universities. In many ways and increasingly, it is better understood that one of the most important missions for AMCs is to create better diagnostics, which are more accurate and contain greater informational content. These better diagnostics would be a tremendous benefit for patients. Furthermore, more effective, less invasive, and more cost-effective therapeutics also can and should be developed. Both challenges have increasingly become the responsibility of AMCs to lead.

Traditionally, AMCs that are able to justify the overhead expense to support a tech transfer function to handle the complexities of IP management. They manage the process of obtaining patent protection and creating license arrangements. These are complex agreements with companies who use those rights to protect their com-

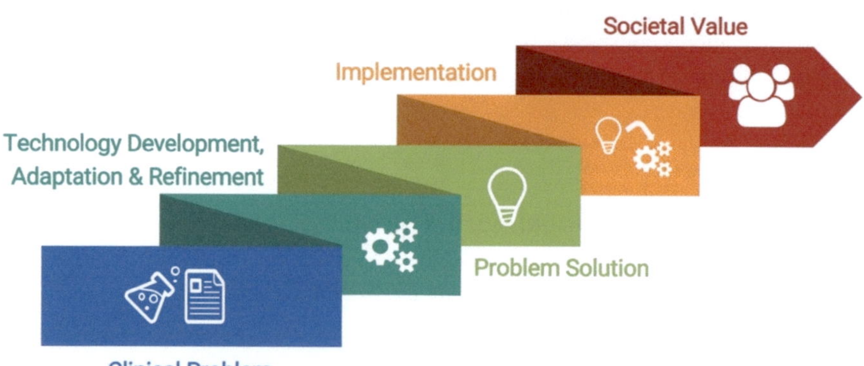

Fig. 15.1 Narrowing the gap between research and clinical translation. Generally, the ideal approach begins with an understanding of the clinical problem with an insightful concept of a step change improvement in the current treatment or diagnostic paradigm. Exploration of technologies that might be refined and/or adapted to enable this invention should follow creating a prototype for a potential solution to the perceived problem. Implementation is complex with staged clinical trials with regulatory implications using the well-developed diagnostic or therapeutic. Ultimately, if the business challenges are overcome, societal value is created, and innovation achieved

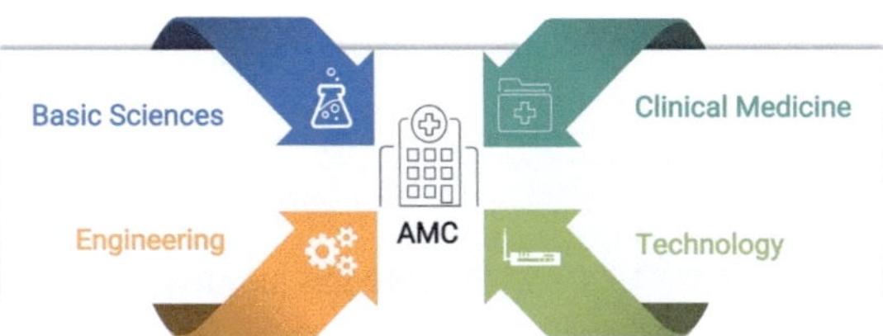

Fig. 15.2 The AMCs benefit from multiple interactions that occur routinely within its hospitable environment. Many of these interactions are leading to an increase in developmental collaboration between clinicians, scientists, engineers, and those within industry. This synergy takes place between the clinicians, who have firsthand knowledge of clinical medicine; the scientists and other investigators, who understand the basic sciences of a disease or disorder; and the engineers and scientists who develop the technologies. Together this can lead to the development of new and adapted innovations that help to overcome those problems previously not conceived. Often multiple of these domains are being addressed by a single individual who possesses both MD and PhD credentials

petitive position after a substantial investment to bring a product through regulatory approval and market introduction, which typically may take many years. Some of the more successful institutions have created a substantial stream of royalty revenue from these licensing activities. Most of those license agreements originate with startup companies who invest the time and capital to create a marketable product [8]. Typically, the new company (NewCo), will then be acquired by an established market player who wishes to acquire the rights to sell the proven innovation through their established product distribution channels.

Dearth of Funding Sources for Translational R&D

A most serious challenge to innovation arises from the dearth of funding available for these early development activities. Although there is generally a tremendous desire to support innovation leading to significant translational successes, it is very uncommon to encounter programs that consistently accomplish these goals. From the investor's perspective, commitment of funding requires trust and an intrinsic faith that the organization they are supporting has the ability and credibility to create commercial value starting from laboratory prototypes and very early model concepts. From the inventor's perspective, it is rare to encounter an environment that supports this freedom to embrace risk and to reach forward to create new paradigms in devices, diagnostics, and therapeutics.

Due to the current risk averse environment particularly in the public domain (i.e. National Institutes of Health), innovation is limited to incremental and often very small advances beyond current state of the art. These advances are frequently inadequate to address the many serious challenges that are encountered in modern medicine. Newer and more effective models are needed to more adequately address this increasing gap.

A New Experiment: Academic Venture Capital

Founding of Partners Innovation Fund

Partners HealthCare System (PHS) was created as an integrated healthcare delivery network anchored by the Massachusetts General Hospital and the Brigham and Women's Hospital. The combined annual research budget exceeds $1.5 billion today generating more than 250 issued patents per year (Fig. 15.3). The technology transfer function was a well-established and high functioning professional operation that returned significant income to the parent organization from its out-licensing activities. An additional critical factor is that the Boston venture capital community is highly developed and productive largely due to the density of sources of IP and technical talent that is the primary driver of any new company created in the life sciences.

The monetization of the invention pipeline in the academic sector has traditionally been limited to early stage licensing of preclinical IP assets. The wealth generated by commercialization of these inventions is largely captured in the form of equity appreciation that benefits the shareholders of these new enterprises founded upon core IP from the AMCs. Tech transfer offices have demonstrated foresight by making share grants part of the financial consideration for license rights packaged with the customary milestone payments and sales royalties [9]. The equity grant is usually small (<10% after first financing) and is subject to dilution in subsequent rounds.

The combined scale of Partners HealthCare System has made it possible to consider non-traditional options to increase the licensor's participation in future product economics. The hospitals have made a decision to expand the tech transfer operation by creating an intramural venture capital function managed by an experienced team of investment professionals. The motivating principle was to join the financing syndicate as co-investor with the same rights, risks, and upside potential that venture capital firms assume when they commit to a new enterprise.

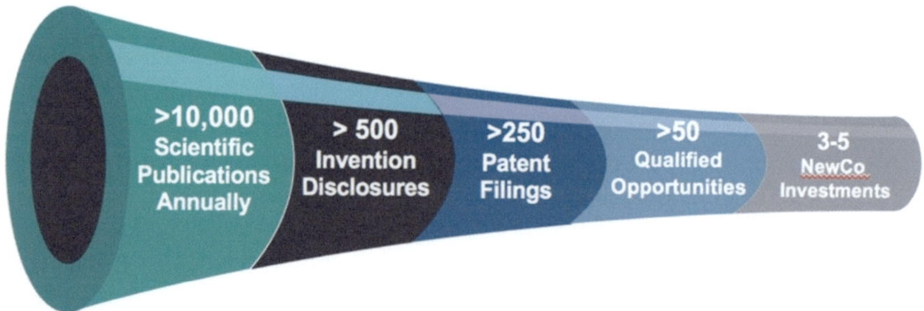

Fig. 15.3 The pipeline of new venture opportunities available to PIF originates from the large knowledge base generated by the PHS investigator community-at-large. The conversion from science to technology to IP to venture creation is a highly reductive process that requires high volume of input to create market worthy innovation

Fund Design, Structure and Operations

Starting with an initial stake of $35 million committed capital, drawn on demand from the hospitals as limited partners, the Partners Innovation Fund (PIF) was incorporated as a Limited Liability Corporation (LLC) in 2008. The fund is governed by a board of managers comprised of the participating hospital CEOs and the system CFO. The fund is strictly limited to consideration of opportunities that contain IP licensed from one or more of the PHS investigator communities.

One of the most important founding principles was to maintain a high standard of objectivity in the evaluation and analysis of investment decisions. The fund management team established a rigorous due diligence process conducted in a manner consistent with standard protocols of the venture capital industry. An external board was established to review all investment recommendations from the fund management team – by this mechanism, decisions are insulated from lobbying forces arising inside the institution. The review board is comprised mostly of executives from the biomedical industry and independent venture capital funds who serve on a *pro bono* basis.

By 2017, PIF had funded more than 30 startups. As expected in the early stage life science sector, there have been more losers than winners across the whole portfolio, but careful risk management continues to deliver highly favorable net returns to date for the hospital limited partners. So much so that the hospitals made the decision to increase their capital commitment and expand the portfolio. Further acknowledging that success, PIF has responded to outside expressions of interest to participate in the investment activities by creating a second fund comprised of investors unrelated to the PHS hospitals, including several major healthcare manufacturers. The second fund, PIF II is managed as a "side car" vehicle by the same management team in tandem with the original core fund. The initial hospital-owned fund was structured as an "evergreen" fund in which dividends, as available, are periodically issued to the limited partner hospitals. PIF II differs in that there is a 10-year lifetime to liquidation, which is the industry standard. The total capital under management has grown to $171 million from the original stake of $35 million.

Relationship with Investigators

PIF recognizes the special nature of its relationship to the hospitals' investigator community. As a "related party", PIF takes responsibility to educate and nurture potential innovators who have no prior experience or training in product development or entrepreneurship. That occurs through specially designed educational outreach programs as well as individual consultation. The goal is to identify homegrown opportunities of high commercial potential and to guide the inventors on a path to successful investment. A form of rubric has been developed that is shared with inventors with the goal to impart an understanding of the thought process by which investors and ultimately customers evaluate new product offerings. Often this reveals a difference of opinion between the inventor and evaluator, but the aim is to bridge understanding and win respect for PIF as a trusted advisor [10].

PIF does not assert any exclusivity on access to IP developed at PHS. Inventors are free to utilize their own connections to pursue their own path to market. The goal of PIF is to serve the system as another option for realizing "return on innovation".

Conflict of Interest Policy and Practice

PHS hospitals are governed by the Harvard University, and particularly the Harvard Medical School, conflict-of-interest policies and these policies also apply to PHS venture fund activities. Hospital faculty and staff inventors who may hold founders as well as investor equity ownership in startups are prohibited from holding simultaneously management positions in their related startups. However, they are allowed to serve as paid consultants, and they may serve on the board of directors under management plans.

Many potential conflicts arise because of interest to further develop IP in the inventor's or investigator's laboratory using funds from the startup or the licensee. If the newly formed company or licensee elects to sponsor research in the investigator's, clinician's, or inventor's laboratory, then a conflict of interest discussion is created. Furthermore, and in addition to the investigator, clinician, or inventor, the institution also can find itself conflicted if the company plans to conduct clinical research at any of the investing hospitals while the fund holds equity in the company or the clinician or inventor plays an active role in this research or its publication. This can be problematic particularly in surgical device development programs when the inventor is often the preferred choice for first clinical deployment of the prototype instruments. These perceived, potential, or real conflicts are currently reviewed and managed by the various PHS hospital or affiliate institution's Committees on Conflict of Interest in collaboration and cooperation with the Harvard Medical School's Standing Committee on Conflict of Interest and Commitment.

Key Lessons Learned

The academic venture fund experiment is in progress, but interim findings can be inferred though not proven. These are some retrospective observations that can be offered for others who are considering their own attempts at institutional venture fund creation.

- To be a successful self-sustaining fund, decisions on investment opportunities must be judged on commercially relevant criteria. External validation should come from objective market-based inquiry into customer value proposition, realistic assessment of product economics, and confirmation from respected co-investors. Despite the relationship that exists between inventor and institution, the investment decision-makers must remember that they are analysts and not advocates.

- Despite their aspirations, inventors are not likely to be the optimal managers for a venture-backed startup. Loss of control to investors is very difficult for inventors to accept but it is the reality of the fundraising process, particularly at the earliest stage of emergence from the AMC laboratories. Professional management trained by the experience of product commercialization is essential to the success of the enterprise.
- It is possible for academic venture funds to maintain a double bottom line of mission and return on investment. A disciplined approach to investment decisions can support the creation of innovations with societal benefits while returning revenue to the host institution for re-investment towards more innovation.

Summary

The potential for AMCs to achieve powerful innovations in twenty-first century healthcare is tremendous given the superb advances made in the physical sciences, genomics, proteomics, metabolomics, imaging medicine, and many other related fields within the last century. The broadening role for AMCs in innovation and development of new devices, diagnostics, and therapeutics has driven an evolved approach in our academic organizations. This shift is moving the field from a risk averse posture, to one that is more supportive and facilitating for translational medicine and its commercialization. The approach by many of the AMCs appears to be expanding from their prior role focused on basic patient care to that of a greater commitment to facilitate invention and innovation for the future of advanced medicine. Many AMCs with a proficient entrepreneurial culture have become actively engaged in the innovation process by not only providing a nurturing entrepreneurial technology transfer environment, but also through exploring their own early venture investment opportunities. These opportunities come not only from simple advisory and collaborative roles, but from ones that provide institutional investment in these new ventures coupled with substantial professional development for the future success of the "NewCo" and/or any inventions. Evolving AMC programs to nurture and grow innovation in the field is critical to creating a better future for patient care, while also supporting the development of clinicians, scientists, and institutions in the twenty-first century of healthcare.

References

1. Sachs G. The digital revolution comes to US healthcare (2015) and centers for disease control heart failure fact sheet.
2. Bayh-Dole Regulations. https://grants.nih.gov/grants/bayh-dole.htm.

 3. Angell M. Is academic medicine for sale? N Engl J Med. 2000;342:1516–8.
 4. Stossel TP. Regulating academic-industrial research relationship—solving problems or stifling progress? N Engl J Med. 2005;353:1060–5.
 5. Loscalzo J. Entrepreneurship in the medical academy: possibilities and challenges in commercialization of research discoveries. Circulation. 2007;115:1504–7.
 6. Moses H, Braunwald E, Martin JB, Thier SO. Collaborating with industry—choices for the academic medical center. N Engl J Med. 2002;347:1371–5.
 7. Toner M, Tompkins RG. Invention, innovation, entrepreneurship in academic medical centers. Surgery. 2008;143:168–71.
 8. Behrns K, Gingles B, Sarr M. Medical innovation - concept to commercialization. 1st ed: Elsevier; 2018. ISBN: 9780128149263
 9. Wong CK, et al. Keys to the kingdom. Nat Biotechnol. 2015;33:232–6.
10. Mas JP, Hseuh B. An investor perspective on forming and funding your medical device startup. Vascular and Interventional Radiology. 2017;20:101–8.

Chapter 16
Training the Next Generation of Surgical Innovators and Entrepreneurs Through a Novel Innovation Pathway and Curriculum

Chandu Vemuri and Mark S. Cohen

Introduction: The Innovation Culture in Academic Surgery and Surgical Training

While much of corporate America has engrained innovation into the fabric of its DNA, the health care sector has shown both a need and fear for innovation resulting in a slower adoption of this culture and its mantras. Creating a true culture of innovation in an academic medical center (AMC) has been a challenge in the past due to the rigors of academic careers, required milestones for faculty and institutions, and limitations stemming from financial concerns or mistrust of developing partnerships with Industry. Fortunately we now live in an age where change, growth, and disruptive technologies are the status quo and the level of advancements in healthcare create a market and competitive atmosphere where development and dissemination of an innovation and entrepreneurial culture are a necessity in order to thrive and compete.

Creating a new culture of innovation in an AMC, though, is no small task as many stakeholders have enjoyed and benefited greatly from the status quo over the years which has focused on research, education, and developing areas of clinical excellence. To this regard, promotion, advancement, and rankings of faculty and academic institutions have been measured using these three pillar missions. Academic faculty and trainees have typically been taught that innovation or entrepreneurship is something you do on the side, if you have time. However growth, consumerism, and competition for patients and their health care dollars has fostered

C. Vemuri
Section of Vascular Surgery, FCVC-5382, Ann Arbor, MI, USA
e-mail: cvemuri@med.umich.edu

M. S. Cohen (✉)
Department of Surgery, University of Michigan, Ann Arbor, MI, USA
e-mail: cohenmar@med.umich.edu

© Springer Nature Switzerland AG 2019

217

M. S. Cohen, L. Kao (eds.), *Success in Academic Surgery: Innovation and Entrepreneurship*, Success in Academic Surgery,
https://doi.org/10.1007/978-3-030-18613-5_16

a need for a competitive advantage in crowded healthcare markets. No longer can the standard academic missions be the only reason patients come to AMCs, but instead patients are now demanding value-based care and the most advanced, cutting edge medical technologies and treatments. This has opened the doors for innovation as a mechanism for AMCs to differentiate themselves from their competition and create new and better treatments for patients. Innovation for many AMCs is now becoming the fourth pillar of academic excellence.

In order to develop an innovation culture in an academic department or institution, as with any culture, this has to start with a shared vision, mission, and buy-in from many stakeholders especially senior leadership all the way down to the most junior faculty, residents, and staff. Once a shared vision for how a department or academic center will embrace and promote innovation, there must be a meaningful mechanism and appropriate resources committed to ensure this can be achieved. Stating a group wants more of their faculty to engage in innovation and entrepreneurship, without giving them time, resources, funding, and incentives for this engagement is a sure set-up for failure. For departments of surgery, in particular, these resources become even more challenging as time spent away from clinical productivity has often a negative impact on the operational bottom line that is needed to keep an organization financially afloat.

What is needed, therefore is development of a meaningful way academic surgeons and trainees can learn to be more effective innovators and translate their solutions into a beneficial impact for their patients. Surgeons are frequently engaged in incorporating new technologies into their practice, where they combine technical skill with creative problem solving to improve tools and techniques. Surgeons are also very sensitive to how health care delivery and patient work flow can affect outcomes and overall costs. What remains a challenge is how to educate surgeons in the area of innovation, commercialization, and entrepreneurship to move their ideas forward in AMCs more effectively. Even surgeons who have had a lifetime of clinical training and experience may lack the necessary tools, skills, and network to successfully take an innovation from an idea to an actual product or service that can impact patient care. The following sections of the chapter will focus on educational methods to train surgeons, and the next generation of trainees and medical students in the art of innovation and entrepreneurship and how this can create a meaningful and sustainable culture in an academic center.

Challenges Educating Surgical Innovators across Different Verticals: Students, Residents, Fellows, Junior and Senior Faculty

Over the past decade, multiple academic institutions have realized the value of education in healthcare innovation. Across institutions and even within institutions the programmatic strategies are varied in part due to variable resources, variable goals, and highly variable target populations. In this section, we will discuss challenges to consider in program design that affect specific trainees as well as general challenges.

Surgical innovation and entrepreneurship has also substantially evolved and is becoming a more viable pathway for academic surgeons to engage in and develop their careers. In fact, several AMCs are now incorporating productivity in innovation and entrepreneurship into their processes for promotion and tenure. As AMCs are trying to bring the newest medical technologies to their patients; practicing surgeons, medical students, resident physicians, and fellows in training are engaging more than ever in the development of novel devices, therapeutics, diagnostics and digital health innovations to improve patient care. How this engagement can effectively occur across different verticals of learners from students to senior faculty will be discussed.

Medical Students and the Need for an Adaptive Innovation Curriculum

Medical School education continues to evolve each year as technology and the breadth of medical knowledge expands. As such, pressures on time and efficiency of learning are at the forefront of training and it has become more and more difficult to add educational content and opportunities into a jam-packed curriculum, especially during the first 2 years of medical school where standard foundational science courses have been shortened to squeeze more content into the curriculum. Yet, these same medical schools are expected to create newly minted and competent physicians after 4 years of education and exposure. In today's medical environment, physicians and especially surgeons must learn to use and evaluate new technologies for their practices putting them on the forefront of current medical technology. Creating meaningful educational content with experiential learning, applying knowledge to real world cases, and solving current medical problems becomes a true challenge in todays medical school curriculum.

While conducting important customer discovery with medical students and faculty, it became evident that there was a significant interest in having opportunities and training for medical students to learn about innovation, design thinking, and commercialization related to medical biotechnologies. Despite this interest there was also a significant concern regarding how much time commitment this opportunity would require as well as the worry that time spent innovating would compete with limited time for classes, exam review, and clerkship experiences. Additionally schedules during daytime hours (8 AM to 5 PM) were relatively packed with lecture, labs, clinical sessions, and simulations. As such several iterations and algorithms were explored over the last several years to create the right mix of foundational and experiential learning to create a meaningful, engaging curriculum in innovation and entrepreneurship for medical students that we have found to be extremely successful and have contributed in a major way to creating a better culture at the medical campus for the clinician innovator.

At the University of Michigan, we have had the fortune of strong institutional support, allowing us to create a longitudinal innovation and entrepreneurship educational program for medical students. The specifics of that program will be discussed below. Medical students are excited to pursue careers with an academic focus in innovation. However, they are a highly varied group from a range of career and educational backgrounds. Therefore they may enter this curriculum with similar enthusiasm in the ideation phase but their ability to translate those ideas into completed projects requires education tailored to their needs. Across the country, medical school curriculum is in continual, rapid evolution. As a result of this, the time that medical students have for extracurricular efforts varies over time and can be unpredictable. This creates a challenge in that structured course content cannot be effectively delivered in a traditional format and for many students, a-la-carte on-line course offerings are more effective, especially for tech-savvy millenials who actively learn through online/digital content everyday. Furthermore, medical students engaging in entrepreneurial activities are often part of a multidisciplinary team and time constraints can complicate an effective meeting schedule of the team. A strategy that can mitigate this can be a digital, on-line platform for content storage, shared calendars and to facilitate interactive meetings. Project execution and exit strategies can also be complex issues for medical students. Most students do not feel comfortable leaving medical school to become a critical member of nascent company and do not have the contacts or time to interview and identify the correct individuals. Lastly medical students have varied clinical interests with minimal clinical expertise, and as such may need a faculty mentor as a functional chief medical officer for their companies. This compounds the logistical complexity of the team as most faculty do not have positions with protected time for healthcare innovation.

Residents

The next level of trainee are residents. In addition to the issues that are involved with medical students, there are unique aspects to training residents in healthcare innovation. As they begin training, residents are more differentiated than students but may not have a final career goal in mind. Layered on top of that is there are a wide variety of training programs with different time requirements, location requirements, and tolerance for non-clinical work during clinical years. During the intense on-service months, residents rarely have the physical time to dedicate to innovation beyond the ideation phase. This can be managed, in part, by leveraging on-line content and on-line platforms for innovation project progression. A key valuable aspect of residency training is academic development time, offered in surgical residencies by many programs. During this time, residents are afforded time away from clinical responsibilities to explore their research and creative interests. Here they may have the time needed for innovation but need mentored, tailored programs to ensure success. These models and paradigms have been developed over decades for basic science and health outcomes research, but funding, space, equipment, intellectual resources and mentorship are less uniformly available across institutions for innovation. Lastly, residents while further along in their training than medical students, still often have limited clinical expertise and will need a dedicated faculty mentor to help with their innovation development clinically.

Fellows

Following residency, many medical and surgical trainees enter rigorous fellowship programs. These programs are nearly always purely clinical and therefore the time issues mentioned above are even more constraining. This group of trainees also needs significant team support and non-traditional educational pathways to be effective innovators. Another unique aspect of fellows is that their time is the shortest of the trainees. They may arrive to an institution and only have 1–2 years. That time frame is sufficient for ideation but project execution with a long-term plan for continued engagement is very difficult to achieve in this shortened period.

Junior Faculty

One of the most exciting developments in academic medicine is the growing interest by junior faculty to learn healthcare innovation as their academic focus. This excitement has been tempered by a significant lack of understanding of the support and resources that are needed to be provided to them by their department to ensure success. Unlike basic science and healthcare sciences, the model of beginning in a mentor's lab with training grants and then progressing to an independent lab with primary grants is not an applicable model at this time in healthcare innovation. Along with this, most faculty interested in innovation are on the clinical track and any time they spend not taking care of patients results in a loss of revenues for their group and employer. Also junior faculty, similar to many trainees, despite having a significant interest in ideation, often lack any relevant training in healthcare innovation and may not have the time to dedicate to a formal training program. Finally, similar to medical students and resident trainees, most faculty are not willing to take the risk of leaving their academic appointments to become critical parts of a start-up and therefore developing start-ups with meaningful exit strategies can be more difficult. Ultimately, with culture change and acceptance of innovation as an important academic pillar, we may reach a future state where successful faculty run funded innovation labs allowing for shared prototyping equipment, critical mentorship and institutional support to provide a meaningful lauching pad for junior faculty to engage in and become successful innovators.

Senior Faculty

In building a culture of innovation and entrepreneurship within a Department of Surgery, one of the more rewarding observations noted was the engagement of senior surgical faculty in surgical innovation opportunities and curriculum. These same individuals who built their careers on developing expertise in research, clinical excellence or teaching, were now seen joining their junior colleagues and applying their natural curiosity and desire to improve patient care and outcomes toward more innovative and entrepreneurial endpoints. Given their deep understanding of the problems in their fields and opportunities to make a meaningful impact for patients allows them to be a vital contributor to the surgical innovation ecosystem. Allowing them to fully engage in the innovative process and join innovation teams with energetic and creative junior faculty, residents, and students adds an important new dimension of diversity to innovation teams and creates significant added value to those teams. In the last 3 years, running three different innovation curricula in the surgery department at the University of Michigan, of the 21 faculty-run teams participating, over 70% of teams had a full professor as an active team member. Of these teams with a senior faculty member engaged as part of the team, 90% were chosen for seed funding >$50,000 each. After completing the innovation courses and curricula, almost all of the senior faculty provided feedback that they had wished they had these types of opportunities to engage in more innovation/entrepreneurial efforts earlier in their careers.

Common Challenges

Across these verticals of learners there are common challenges to be addressed. Programs need to be tailored as traditional training programs will not be attended and therefore a wasted effort. Significant funding sources need to exist and innovators need to be made aware of their existence to support ideas beyond the innovation phase. Physical innovation spaces are needed to allow for meetings but also to provide resources for prototyping equipment, collaboration opportunities and streamlined access to intellectual resources. A common challenge to innovation programs is project execution. Due to the factors discussed above this will require unique collaborative agreements, multi-disciplinary teams, and pre-made contracts specifying future returns and exit strategies based on longitudinal contributions. Understanding these challenges across the various groups is key to creating successful innovation programs.

A Path of Excellence in Innovation and Entrepreneurship for Medical Students

Recognizing the growing need for medical students to understand how to develop and better interface with the growing number of medical innovations emerging into the market and pre-market studies each year, it becomes vital for medical schools to offer more formalized training in this area. In order to meet the needs of a wide variety of learners from gen Z, millenials, all the way to baby boomers who all learn a bit differently, resources for innovation and educational opportunities need to be adaptable for trainees to have meaningful participation and engagement. To meet this need, we utilized experiential learning, digital media platforms, and reversed classroom opportunities to optimize engagement and interest from such a diverse group.

In addition to the creating a strong foundational education that helps students identify and solve the right problems in medicine and use iterative design thinking mixed with customer discovery to de-risk and develop a strong value proposition, medical schools wanting a sustainable effort in Innovation and Entrepreneurship must also commit financial resources toward trainee and project development. These resources are critical to establishing and sustaining the innovation culture, but often the hardest resource to allocate at major academic medical centers is time for trainees and students to engage fully in innovation efforts, discovery, and development. For most students and trainees, time is very limited for these innovation activities, which have been marginalized as "extracurricular" at best at most centers. Recognizing the importance of innovation in medicine for the future and the critical need for resources to support medical students, residents, and faculty in this innovation and entrepreneurial development, we embarked on the programmatic development of a innovation and entrepreneurship curriculum for medical learners that recognizes some unique challenges for medical technologies compared to other business sectors.

In 2015, a survey was conducted to the first-year medical school class of 170 students at the University of Michigan, asking whether students wished to participate in a 4-year co-curricular pathway in Innovation and Entrepreneurship to develop their ideas and learn more about this area for their future careers. Thirty-five percent responded they would participate in such a path, and this was a big catalyst that lead to the development of the first "Pathway of Excellence (PoE) in Innovation and Entrepreneurship (I&E)" being created and approved by the medical school curriculum committee for implementation later that year. One goal of the I&E PoE was to incorporate relevant and high-yield content, infrastructure, and opportunities already developed by other innovation programs in the Engineering School and the Business School and add to these the unique aspects and challenges that medical technologies and industries must navigate in order to create meaningful impact for patients.

The Pathway of Excellence in Innovation and Entrepreneurship (I&E) was approved in the fall of 2015 and in its inaugural year, admitted 31 first year medical students and nine students from the second or third year medical school classes. Its core mission is to provide physicians-in-training the resources, perspective, and exposure they need to incorporate innovative strategies and tools that can improve the quality and equity of medical care. An important goal of the I&E PoE is to develop medical students who can understand how to address real medical problems and patient needs through medical innovation and entrepreneurial solutions and explore the transformational role physician-innovators have on health care.

Curricular Development and Offerings for the PoE in Innovation and Entrepreneurship:

In constructing the educational/curricular portion of the Innovation PoE, many moving parts of the complex medical school curriculum had to be traversed. In fact the medical school curriculum had major changes every year for the last 3 years forcing the I&E curriculum to be flexibile and adaptive to this changing medical school educational environment. As such, a lot of thought had to be put into how to build flexibility into the learning infrastructure so that it could be utilized effectively by students and trainees with limited time constraints. For example, a standard semester or year long didactic course while traditional for many business schools, would not be effective or attended in this environment. In the first year of the curriculum, a year-long course in innovation was developed for residents and fellows through the Fast Forward Medical Innovation group and it was called the PACE (Program to Accelerate Commercialization Education) course. This evening course over two semesters was built upon many of the principles of I-Corps (training in business development and customer discovery provided to small businesses from the National Institute of Health and National Science Foundation) but then enhanced with content unique for medical technologies such as hospital economics, CMS approval, purchasing, and DRG/CPT coding and reimbursement. While the course was offered to the initial I&E PoE students, their attendance was sparce and sporadic due to time constraints from their other medical school classes and commitments.

To address these time constraints for students, the content of the PACE course was then in the following year adapted and condensed to shortened, high yield topics focused on customer discovery, value proposition development, and understanding the key components of a compelling pitch. Additional foundational material was put into digital format including online modules with self assessment on Intellectual Property, regulatory pathways, clinical trials, FDA, prototyping, design thinking, funding strategies, stakeholder analysis, licensing and startup ventures, and more. In addition to the online modules and guest faculty and alumni lectures, the medical school committed several blocks of dedicated pathway time during the day throughout the academic year to allow interface of pathway content with students. During this time, a more engaging reversed-classroom model was utilized to evaluate real world cases and pick apart issues with value proposition, customer discovery, and business approach models. Real clinician-entrepreneurs were also brought in from strategic companies as well as smaller startups to talk about their challenges and how they navigated their environment to become successful, or their failures and why they failed. Students were each paired with faculty mentors and innovation advisors to help them think through their own innovation ideas, and work together on multidisciplinary teams often with engineers, MBA students, law students, or with other medical students and faculty.

Once students completed this basic fundamental core curriculum, they then work on developing a mentored capstone project. Each capstone is unique and designed by the student with their advisors and mentors to explore more fully an innovation or commercial opportunity of their interest. Students are encouraged to engage with faculty mentors, participate in internships and externships with faculty, local startups, VC firms, bigger strategic companies in medical device, therapeutics, or diganostics, as well with our Fast Forward Medical Innovation group at the medical center to work on due diligence and milestone achievement of University funded projects in this space. Currently all graduating medical students are required to complete a dedicated capstone project for clinical impact, and I&E PoE students can complete this graduation requirement through their innovation pathway capstone project. Over the last 3 years, students participating in the PoE have successfully spun out over 12 start-up companies, with several acquiring substantial investment follow-on funding. A few students have been given the opportunity to take a year off from medical school to run their new company as CEO and really understand the challenges of running a startup. Others have pursued combined MD/MBA degrees (with the number of students seeking this dual degree more than doubling since the PoE was created).

This ecosystem of mentor-mentee relationships for innovation within the university has been a critical component to developing a new culture among medical students that supports and promotes innovation and entrepreneurship. With every department of the medical school participating in these innovation programs across the medical campus, students have the great benefit of working with a diverse group of faculty innovators as well as a larger, more diverse pool of medical innovation projects. This has helped to create an ideal culture and environment to train the next generation of medical innovators for success [1, 2].

Beyond the PoE offerings, the medical school also has a number of extracurricular groups that offer greater opportunities to explore innovation. The Medical Innovation Group (MIG) along with other groups on campus including the summer Surgery SCRUBS program helped create a medical student Shark Tank competition program. This was an 8-month incubator program for teams of medical students to create innovative healthcare ideas around surgical problems. The program culminated in a "Shark Tank" style finale in which teams competed in front of seasoned venture capitalists and entrepreneurs for Medical School-funded seed-grants. Simultaneously, the medical school fully supported the founding of a Michigan chapter of SLING Health (formerly IDEA labs). This is a student-run organization focused on developing multidisciplinary biodesign teams (combining medical, engineering, business, and law students) to address healthcare solutions. SLING Health provides resources, early funding, mentorship, engineering design review evaluations, prototype development, and a DEMO-Day competition in a Shark-Tank style format where the winning teams are sponsored to attend the national SLING Health DEMO-Day where the best innovations from each of the SLING programs across the country compete for funding awards.

One of the challenges with any of the courses or curricula that were offered through the medical campus, whether they were for students, faculty, or residents, was that participants comprised a fairly homogenous group in the same specialty or training level. While this provides some diversity of thought, it is harder to generate the truly disruptive ideas that real innovation diversity can bring. There is also a challenge or problem with creating courses attended by a diverse group of faculty and students from multiple fields and schools in that coordination, funding of tuition across schools, and lack of alignment with schedules is difficult to navigate.

To solve this problem, a collaboration between the I&E PoE, the Center For Entrepreneruship at the Engineering School, FFMI, and MBAs at the Business School was forged to create the Medical Innovators Pitch Club (MI-PITCH CLUB). The vision and purpose of MI-PITCH is to organically bring together engineers, medical professionals, finance and business professionals, public health experts, scientists, and policy experts to network regularly and solve REAL MEDICAL PROBLEMS faced on campus. Together this diverse group of innovators develop solutions each month that not only help patients locally but can also translate to help patients nationally and even globally.

One KEY difference between MI-PITCH and other types of "PITCH CLUBS" put together by VC groups or local tech-groups is that the goal of MI-PITCH is not to just bring in start-ups to practice pitching their technologies and getting feedback on their pitches. While there is opportunity for faculty and students who come to MI-PITCH to practice pitching their new ideas and build broader multidisciplinary teams around their ideas or get important customer discovery and feedback during the networking hour each session, the main DIFFERENTIATOR of MI-PITCH is that each month, a different department, center or group sponsors the event and creates the medical design challenge for the month. What this means is that a real medical problem that could be solved by a device, diagnostic, process improvement, algorithm, or digital health solution is presented to the group. The presenter from the sponsoring department or group provides the medical problem being faced, defines the current pains and gains to stakeholders related to the problem and current solutions, and then poses the real question they would like addressed by the MI-PITCH audience. The audience then pairs up into teams of 3–4 people including medical, engineering, and business professionals on each team and works on a solution to the problem to define their value proposition and implementation of their solution to the audience and judges.

The benefit to the sponsoring department or group is they then get 50–100 highly innovative people from multiple backgrounds (medical professionals, engineers, and MBAs) working in multidisciplinary teams to come up with a design solution to the problem including a value proposition, a model/prototype/ drawing/algorithm, and a basic cost/revenue justification for a business case. The sponsor/department can then take these creative solutions and decide if they want to invest additional seed money to advance the project further and then apply for bigger internal funding opportunities. This process organically create new networks and partnerships and has already engaged over 400 people18 in its first six months running from 6 schools and 19 departments on campus.

Training Residents, Fellows and Junior Faculty in Innovation & Entrepreneurship

Just as team science is transforming traditional research, team innovation is necessary for success. Any given individual will not have all of the talent required to take a project from ideation to successful execution. We believe it is useful to have a few different team models based on categories of innovation including information technology, process improvement, medical devices, and drugs. For example, a medical device team may need a mechanical/electrical/biomaterials engineer whereas a process improvement team may need industrial engineers. Therefore it is critical to create teams with the intellectual resources needed for successful project development. It is also important to consider time constraints, team member abilities and availability, and exit strategies when creating teams.

As with any educational program, coaching and mentorship are absolutely critical. Identifying mentors who are specifically interested in creating a culture of healthcare innovation and who have the time, physical resources, money, and experience to guide young innovators through project cycles is paramount. Furthermore, mentors are needed from multiple schools including engineering, medicine, business, and law.

Innovation programs could be designed in the model of a startup with an initial investment of time, money, space, and equipment. In that model success may be measured in publications, patents, companies created, and financial return on investment. There are several program components that are needed to achieve success. First there must be a clear program to guide project management, to ensure project development, and then to guarantee execution. This will require physical resources such as dedicated space for meetings, prototyping equipment, as well as software and project managers to guide groups along their commercialization pathways. Additionally the core concepts of customer discovery, identifying regulatory guidance, studying the intellectual property landscape, creating a business model, and the ability to rapidly and cheaply prototype must all be taught to learners. Additionally key intellectual and physical resources must be present and readily accessible to teams. The project manager must teach teams how to fail early and how to rapidly pivot to meet the needs and demands of the market and the customer. Teams also need guidance creating project specific key performance indicators (KPIs) as well and program specific KPIs. These KPIs must be designed to ensure a meaningful return on investment for the innovation program and to meet local, regional, and national metrics for success. Lastly, innovation programs must use non-traditional novel teaching techniques. Simply put self-directed learning tools, on-line courses, and 24/7 access to intellectual resources has become a requirement in todays fast paced learning environment. This will require the development of customer driven websites with high-quality, tailored content accessible across a variety of mobile and fixed platforms.

Moving Technologies out of the University

Unlike corporations, universities need to have clear, accessible, defined, and funded pathways for moving successful technologies out into the private sector. In our institution the tech transfer office provides key support in working through patent applications, exploring intellectual property landscapes, LLC filings, corporate structure, licensing, and other common commercialization processes. Equally important to this effort is to have an organized database of seed funding and business development contacts with an intentional, easy mechanism for teams to get in front of these contacts to be heard, funded, and advanced.

Examples of Student/Resident/Faculty Team Programs and Technologies

Our institution has multiple healthcare innovation programs. In this section we will highlight a few innovation teams funded by the University of Michigan Department of Surgery and others by the Frankel Cardiovascular Center.

The University of Michigan Department of Surgery through the Michigan Promise has made a commitment to foster surgical innovation. One of the big programs of the Michigan Promise is the Michigan Surgical Innovation Prize Program.

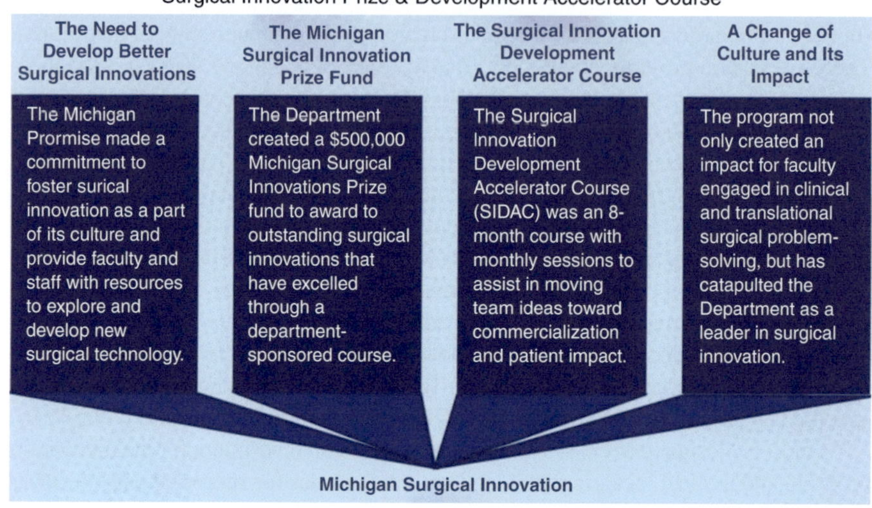

Source: https://medicine.umich.edu/dept/surgery/news/archive/201810/surgical-innovation-prize-development-accelerator-course

The Michigan Surgical Innovation Prize Fund

In 2016, the Department of Surgery at the University of Michigan ran its first Surgical Innovation and Entrepreneurship Development Program (SIEDP) where 13 surgery faculty (from new assistant professors to senior leadership in the department) participated in a 9 month training program where they had sessions 1 day per month covering the commercialization process from idea generation all the way to technology development, patent submission, customer discovery, funding, and implementation. All of the faculty in the program participated on teams and learned this process culminating in a "final pitch" grand-rounds, which was done in a Shark-Tank style where industry experts and Venture Capital partners outside the University could evaluate the technologies more thoroughly. One of the key departmental projects produced from the SIEDP was a Department Sponsored Contract Research Organization (CRO) (*https://medicine.umich.edu/dept/surgery/news/archive/*

201810/surgical-innovation-prize-development-accelerator-course) to connect big industry and startup companies with faculty labs to set up contract projects that utilize the unique research tools available in the Department. This project has now resulted in several new industry contracts that brought in additional revenues to the Department's diverse research funding portfolio and currently provides engaged faculty labs with additional support for high-risk/high reward research. (J. Surg Ed 2018; 75(4). 936–941) [3].

In addition to generating great surgical innovation projects, the course provided key knowledge and resources to the participating surgical faculty, allowing them the time and ability to pursue their innovation interests in a protected environment. Through this course and process, many have gone on to be serial innovators and have engaged other innovation resources around the campus (such as Fast Forward Medical Innovation, NIH SBIR, and Coulter Funding Programs). This has created a wonderful cultural evolution in the Department where surgical innovation and entrepreneurship have now become part of the groups academic DNA and core mission, where faculty innovators are seen as individuals worth supporting and recognizing within the Department. This departmental commitment to fostering and enhancing its innovation culture, lead to the vision and creation of the Michigan Surgical Innovation Prize Fund. Through this fund, within the Michigan Promise, the Department created a $500,000 Michigan Surgical Innovation Prize fund awarding outstanding surgical innovations that have excelled through a department-sponsored Surgical Innovation Development Accelerator Course (SIDAC). The Michigan Surgical Innovation Prize is the first of its kind in the country and its mission is to foster and accelerate the development of novel technologies that will improve surgical diseases or the care of surgical patients. The first round of the $500,000 prize was awarded in August 2018 and split between 6 outstanding surgical innovation technologies lead by core faculty in the department.

The Surgical Innovation Development Accelerator Course

In August of 2017, a request for proposals for the first Michigan Surgical Innovation Prize was sent out across the Medical School and the School of Engineering. Each proposal had to address a surgical problem or disease with an innovation or solution that improves the lives of surgical patients. These innovations could be in the form of new devices, diagnostics, therapeutics, digital health solutions, or programmatic efforts, but all had to be translatable into real patient/commercial impact. Multidisciplinary collaborative team projects were encouraged as long as a surgery faculty member was actively involved. Over 30 outstanding proposals were submitted into the competition in the form of an executive summary. Each was reviewed, discussed, and ranked by our innovation prize oversight committee, made up of faculty experts in and out of the department, along with engineering, regulatory, and legal IP experts, industry leaders, and venture capital partners to assure content expertise, oversight and expert diligence regarding funding decisions and the proper use of funds.

From this cohort of applications, 12 finalist teams were picked to participate in the newly updated Surgical Innovation Development Accelerator Course (SIDAC), which was run by a lead instructor who was a serial entrepreneur. This was an eight-month course (January–August 2018) with once monthly all-day sessions set up to assist teams in moving their ideas toward commercialization and patient impact. Each team had expert instruction, guided expert mentorship and coaching, as well as peer mentorship and coaching from others in the course, and resources for patent filing, prototyping, and customer discovery provided through the fund and supported by the Office of Technology Transfer (https://techtransfer.umich.edu) and the Fast Forward Medical Innovation group (https://innovation.medicine.umich.edu). SIDAC taught teams the following concepts: idea generation, value proposition, intellectual property and patent submission, regulatory pathways, customer discovery, marketing and adoption, reimbursement and funding models, prototyping and pitching. The teams all worked on advancing their technologies through the course and in August 2018 they provided their updated executive summaries of their technologies and pitched their ideas to the oversight committee for questions and evaluation. Of the finalist teams presenting to the OC, 6 of the teams had technologies advanced and derisked enough to warrant a combined $480,000 of funding through the Michigan Surgical innovation Prize. The top four teams then pitched their innovations in front of the entire department and three guest Sharks (two venture capital senior partners and a physician innovator and academic chair) at a Shark Tank-style Grand Rounds. (https://www.youtube.com/watch?v=eQzcQV6YzOs&feature=youtu.be).

Some thoughts from our SIDAC participants include:

"It's a real testimony to the Department of Surgery to allow their faculty to explore these interests which inherently have value to our patients, getting innovations from our brains to the bedside."

"It's nice to sit in a room with a bunch of other people doing the same thing because they all have really helpful suggestions for your own idea. It's interesting to hear about the processes they have gone through and the kinds of resources that they've used because those are often helpful for your own project."

"This is a fantastic program in regards to mentoring, because you have different levels and different kinds of mentorship ... In this space, you really need mentorship from engineering, you need mentorship from lawyers, you need mentorship from people who understand customer exploration, people who understand prototyping."

Winners of the FIRST Michigan Surgical Innovation Prize Competition August 2018 [4–7]

Ferroximend - A novel therapeutic device for bone healing

Ferroximend combines an angiogenic stimulant, deferoxamine, with an osteogenic (bone forming) tissue filler device, hyaluronic acid. This unique combination triggers the formation of blood vessels at the fracture site, at the right time, leading to a remarkable ability to heal difficult fractures and accelerate that healing process.

Michigan ENdoluminal lengthening Device (MEND)

MEND is a device technology therapy that uses the well-established medical principle of mechanotrasduction to induce growth of new intestine and is intended to safely treat short bowel syndrome unlike current available therapy.

"In order for these things to move forward it goes beyond the normal skill set that we learn as a professor or as a doctor. It puts you in a different mindset and it's leading to very fruitful outcomes."

Minute Coaching System

The minute coaching system is a proprietary software product that lets medical students get real time feedback from faculty. The goal is to sell/license this product out to other medical schools, either directly from University of Michigan or via an existing company with a franchise in the medical education market.

"Part of the innovation prize is to help us figure out a way to make this applicable to a broader group of people. So can we take our feedback system, and can we make it financially viable and something that we can create into a product that could be used for other departments within the med school, other universities, other Departments of Surgery?"

Surgical Asset Tracker

Surgical Asset Tracker is a University of Michigan startup that develops and commercializes software solutions for tracking temporary implantable devices, providing automated, high fidelity device-tracking with alerts and works with any major EHR.

"I think it's easy to invent things, and ideas come easily to many of us, but there's a huge gap between the idea and actually making something that'll impact patients, and I think, as a physician or a scientist, we don't have a lot of knowledge about that gap, about markets and how to actually bring things to them, so this fills that gap."

Hot Spot - Using Thermochromic Material to Identify Areas at Risk for Ulcer

This technology uses thermochromic liquid crystals that change color providing an obvious, early warning sign that patients may be at risk for ulcer formation.

"We were learning all about how to present a business plan, how to present our ideas, and really working closely with the innovation department here to come up with strategies of how to market our device. And this was a lot of work over the past nine months with our team but I think we learned a lot along the way and came up with a great presentation."

MULT-EYE Laparoscopic Camera

A multi-camera based integrated imaging system for improved visualization during laparoscopic surgery.

Next Steps for the Program

Teams funded through the program will now use their award money toward advancing their technologies to meaningful impact for surgical patients in a timeline and milestone-based format. Funded teams will continue to meet with their mentors/ coaches and provide updates to the oversight committee twice a year with a formal update presentation session next year in August 2019. Teams are also eligible and encouraged to apply for other funding mechanisms within the University (Through FFMI or the Coulter Program as well as through the Center for Entrepreneurship) as well as outside the University (National SBIR/STTR funding from NIH or NSF). After 9 months of follow-up since their MSIP awards, teams have already won an additional $450,000 in follow-on funding with more coming in by the end of the year.

The next request for proposals for our second Round of the $500,000 Surgical Innovation Prize will be opened in August of 2019 with the goal of increasing the prize value and program resources through individual and industry collaboration and support.

Michigan Surgical Innovation Accelerator Program

Given the amazing success of the first round of the Michigan Surgical Innovation Prize, to continue this momentum as well as develop winning team projects for the next round in 2019, an opportunity was created (during the off year between rounds of the big Surgical Innovation Prize Competition) for surgical innovation teams who are early in their technology development to accelerate and de-risk their ideas through expert education/coaching/mentorship and customer discovery. This $100,000 accelerator funded 5 promising surgical technologies to move through a custom commercialization program over 6 months intended to advance these technologies to a point where they will be highly competitive for follow-on funding. Technologies again had to address a solution to a surgical problem and benefit/ advance the care of surgical patients and a Department of Surgery full time faculty must be the PI or co-PI on the project. Teams each received 14 hours of didactic education, 20 hours of 1-on-1 coaching and expert mentorship, as well as opportunities to complete 30 customer discovery interviews, a regulatory roadmap assessment from a contracted and trusted regulatory development agency, as well as funding to complete basic prototyping for devices. Additional funding was available for travel for additional customer discovery and any killer experiments needed to derisk the technology and advance it along its regulatory pathway. Winning Projects included: RETREVA – a novel laparascopic retrieval device for limited volume locations; "My weight loss journey": A novel bariatric surgery companion digital application; a synthetic polymer scaffold niche for early detection of metastatic breast cancer; using mobile technology to detect patients having a stroke; and a "Continuous Non-Invasive Monitoring of End-organ Cellular Function with Super-Continuum Laser Spectroscopy". Each of these technologies has now been de-risked and advanced in house to be competetive for the next big Michigan Surgical Innovation Prize.

A Change of Culture and Its Impact

The last 3 years have demonstrated numerous successful programs and resources for faculty in Innovation and Entrepreneurship across the University of Michigan medical campus and the MSIP/SIDAC program in the Department of Surgery is one of the more advanced and tailored programs of this group and unique among Departments of Surgery in the world. The success and impact from this program in innovation has stimulated change in other departments on the medical campus, leading other departments and centers to engage in their own innovation efforts. Together this has created a broader impact on the academic culture at the University of Michigan, where "Innovation" has now become one of the core values of Michigan Medicine. Through this transformative first Michigan Surgical Innovation Prize Competition and SIDAC course, over 40 surgeons, scientists, engineers, surgical residents, and medical students gained critical knowledge of the value and development of surgical technologies toward patient use and impact. These participants now understand how cultivate diverse teams and to navigate their ideas through the university as well as beyond into the market. The program has not only created tremendous impact within the Department for faculty engaged in clinical and translational surgical problem-solving, but has catapulted Michigan's Department of Surgery as a national leader in Surgical Innovation.

Frankel Cardiovascular Center (FCVC) Innovation Program and Aikens Innovation Academy

This new program was created to create value in cardiovascular healthcare through innovation. Similar to the Michigan Surgical Innovation Prize and the SIDAC program, the FCVC Innovation Program structure includes a pitch event and then a year-long custom educational program to ensure that funded teams complete their projects. This program is unique in that the teams can be from any staff member of the FCVC such as medical professionals (physicians, nurses, advanced practice providers), industrial engineers and check in staff.

The 2018–2019 program funded the following teams: preventing deconditioning of heart failure patients while they are in our hospitals and after discharge, routine grip strength measurement for frailty screening in cardiovascular clinics, post intensive cardiac care outpatient long term outreach clinic for survivors of the cardiac intensive care unit and a virtual reality tool to the simulation the MRI experience. As a reflection of the diverse group of applicants, these teams included medical and non-medical staff and are largely focused on process improvement, which can be applied quickly to impacting patient care in a meaningful and direct way.

References and Links

1. Cohen MS. Enhancing surgical innovation through a specialized medical school pathway of excellence in innovation and entrepreneurship: Lessons learned and opportunities for the future. Surgery. 2017;162:989–93.
2. Cohen MS. Innovation series. In: Surgery; 2018. pii: S0039–6060(18)30492–6.
3. Servoss J, Chang C, Olson D, Ward KR, Mulholland MW, Cohen MS. The Surgery Innovation and Entrepreneurship Development Program (SIEDP): an experiential learning program for surgery faculty to ideate and implement innovations in health care. J Surg Educ. 2018;75(4):935–41.
4. Michigan Surgery Shark Tank Videos: https://www.youtube.com/watch?v=eQzcQV6YzOs&feature=youtu.be
5. Office of Technology Transfer. https://techtransfer.umich.edu
6. Fast Forward Medical Innovation group. https://innovation.medicine.umich.edu
7. https://medicine.umich.edu/dept/surgery/news/archive/201810/surgical-innovation-prize-development-accelerator-course

Index